T0323756

"Stefani Goerlich and Elyssa Helfer skillfully write about the misunderstood topic of kink and BDSM with much clarity, dispelling the myths and harmful assumptions, and making this book an accessible and enjoyable read. This book is well researched and includes all the complexities and nuances of kink and BDSM, from pleasure and pain to benefits and risks. It is a must-read for all therapists and other professionals in becoming kink-informed and kink-affirmative."

Silva Neves, *author of* Sexology: The Basics

"*BDSM and Kink: The Basics* is a thorough exploration of kink that is much needed, for both those who want to explore their own sexuality and those who want to understand kinky people. The only way to combat the stigma around these sexual practices and marginalized communities is through frank discussion and education about consent and the skills that are needed to play safely. Every professional should also understand these dynamics to better assist their clients who are kinky."

Susan Wright, *National Coalition for Sexual Freedom*

BDSM AND KINK: THE BASICS

BDSM and Kink: The Basics provides an essential overview of knowledge that every clinician should have about alternative sexualities.

In an accessible, user-friendly format, the authors offer a high-level yet comprehensive introduction to the world of bondage and discipline, dominance and submission, sadomasochism, fetishists, and more. Written by two of the leading experts on working with kinky clients, *BDSM and Kink: The Basics* takes a sex-positive, kink-affirming approach to the material, exploring everything from etiologies and basic terminology through risk assessment and clinical best practices. The perfect desk reference for any clinician who wants to expand their understanding of erotic minorities, this book will prepare you to meet your clients with curiosity and competency while offering digital resources and specific suggestions to deepen your knowledge wherever you need it most.

This book is essential for mental health and medical providers, educators, and individuals interested in learning more about BDSM and kink.

Stefani Goerlich is the multi-award-winning author of three books on BDSM/kink and mental health. She is a sex therapist, lecturer, forensic consultant, and co-host of the *Securing Sexuality* podcast.

Elyssa Helfer is a sex therapist specializing in working with the BDSM/kink community. She is an adjunct professor, research associate, and fierce advocate for sexual freedom.

The Basics Series

The Basics is a highly successful series of accessible guidebooks which provide an overview of the fundamental principles of a subject area in a jargon-free and undaunting format.

Intended for students approaching a subject for the first time, the books both introduce the essentials of a subject and provide an ideal springboard for further study. With over 50 titles spanning subjects from artificial intelligence (AI) to women's studies, *The Basics* are an ideal starting point for students seeking to understand a subject area.

Each text comes with recommendations for further study and gradually introduces the complexities and nuances within a subject.

BDSM AND KINK
Stefani Goerlich and Elyssa Helfer

SIMONE DE BEAUVOIR
Megan Burke

INTERVIEWING: THE BASICS
Mark Holton

SHAKESPEARE (FOURTH EDITION)
Sean McEvoy

DREAMS
Dale Mathers and Carola Mathers

For a full list of titles in this series, please visit www.routledge.com/The-Basics/book-series/B

BDSM AND KINK

THE BASICS

Stefani Goerlich and Elyssa Helfer

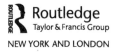

NEW YORK AND LONDON

Designed cover image: Pink leather texture background © kumpolstock/Getty Images

First published 2025
by Routledge
605 Third Avenue, New York, NY 10158

and by Routledge
4 Park Square, Milton Park, Abingdon, Oxon, OX14 4RN

Routledge is an imprint of the Taylor & Francis Group, an informa business

© 2025 Stefani Goerlich and Elyssa Helfer

Library of Congress Cataloging-in-Publication Data
Names: Goerlich, Stefani, author. | Helfer, Elyssa, author.
Title: BDSM and kink : the basics / Stefani Goerlich and Elyssa Helfer.
Description: New York, NY : Routledge, 2025. | Series: The basics |
    Includes bibliographical references and index.
Identifiers: LCCN 2024020528 (print) | LCCN 2024020529 (ebook) |
    ISBN 9781032321028 (hardback) | ISBN 9781032320632 (paperback) |
    ISBN 9781003312833 (ebook)
Subjects: LCSH: Bondage (Sexual behavior)—Psychological aspects. | Sex therapy. |
    Sexual dominance and submission—Psychological aspects. | Sex (Psychology) |
    Fetishism (Sexual behavior)
Classification: LCC HQ79 .G625 2025 (print) | LCC HQ79 (ebook) |
    DDC 306.77—dc23/eng/20240531
LC record available at https://lccn.loc.gov/2024020528
LC ebook record available at https://lccn.loc.gov/2024020529

ISBN: 978-1-032-32102-8 (hbk)
ISBN: 978-1-032-32063-2 (pbk)
ISBN: 978-1-003-31283-3 (ebk)

DOI: 10.4324/9781003312833

Typeset in Bembo
by Apex CoVantage, LLC

To those who have come before me and those who fight alongside me; may every step we take bring us closer to the world we dream of.

E.H.

To Amanda and Brittany, For your solidarity, support, and shenanigans.

To my Wolf, forever.

S.G.

CONTENTS

List of Figures   xi
List of Tables   xii
Acknowledgments   xiii

1 **What Is Kink?**   1
   Stefani Goerlich

2 **Bondage and Discipline**   15
   Stefani Goerlich

3 **Dominance and Submission**   36
   Elyssa Helfer

4 **Sadomasochism**   52
   Stefani Goerlich

5 **Power Exchange Roleplay**   77
   Elyssa Helfer

6 **Fetishes**   89
   Stefani Goerlich

7 **What Does a Kinky Scene Look Like?**   103
   Elyssa Helfer

8 **Problematic Behavior**   124
   Elyssa Helfer

9   **Assessing Risk and Safety**   **152**
    Stefani Goerlich

10 **Best Practices for Working with Kinky Clients**   **175**
    Elyssa Helfer

Conclusion   191
Bibliography   193
Index   211

FIGURES

2.1 Decorative *Shibari* (QR code)   18
2.2 Mechanical Bondage (QR code)   20
3.1 Kinkly Sex Terms (QR code)   46
4.1 The Science of BDSM Research (QR code)   55
4.2 Swami Temple Kavadi (QR code)   56
6.1 Short HarmonyX Documentary (QR code)   99
6.2 The *Securing Sexuality* Podcast (QR code)   101
7.1 The Alternative Sexualities Health Research
    Alliance (TASHRA) (QR code)   107
7.2 The National Coalition for Sexual Freedom
    (NCSF) (QR code)   107
7.3 The Science of BDSM Lab (QR code)   108
7.4 The Community-Academic Consortium for Research
    on Alternative Sexualities (CARAS) (QR code)   109
7.5 Kink and Scene Negotiation (QR code)   114
8.1 Sex FAQs & Information from the Kinsey
    Institute (QR code)   127
8.2 Paraphilic Disorders   143
10.1 Kink Clinical Guidelines (QR code)   182

TABLES

1.1   An Incomplete Taxonomy of Kink   7

ACKNOWLEDGMENTS

There are so many people in my life who have been a part of this unexpected journey with me; so many pillars of support who deserve far more than a few words on a page. That said, I will never pass up the opportunity to shout your praises from any and all spaces that are available to me. I cannot acknowledge anyone without first expressing my deepest gratitude to my co-author, Stefani. Without your trust and belief in me, I would not be here. Not only did you invite me into your world, you opened the door with no expectation of me to be anything other than myself. You've given me a gift—one that I will cherish for the rest of my life. To my family: it is challenging to put into words my gratitude to you all. I know that a part of loving me means never knowing which direction I will go in next. You never doubt me; you never dissuade me; you do nothing but support me. How I got this lucky, I'll never know. To my incredible friends, Joslyn Bronson, Brandon McCourt, Hillary Nadworny, Lauren Talaga, Danielle Kramer, and Sarah Limcaco: I simply could not be me without you. To my mentors, Richard Sprott and Anna Randall: I will never be able to adequately thank you for taking a chance on me. Your unwavering dedication, passion, and sacrifices do not go unnoticed. You inspire me always.

To my therapist, Kate Loree: many years ago, you presented two roads in front of me—two different futures that required me to make a difficult and lifechanging choice. To show up in my truth or to keep hiding from it. You helped set me free. And lastly, to my partner, Frank Mons: you were the first to add fuel to my fire. You make the seemingly impossible feel possible. You are everything.

Elyssa Helfer, PhD

WHAT IS KINK?
Stefani Goerlich

INTRODUCTION

This is a book about relationships. The relationships people have with their bodies. The relationships people have with their environments. And the relationships people have with one another. Often, when we approach the topic of BDSM and kink, we assume that the subject is sexual, prurient, deviant, explicit. Indeed, we often see kink portrayed in popular culture as a form of sexual expression—and it certainly can be. But it is first and foremost a relational expression—a way of cultivating and maintaining emotional and sensory connections between the kinky person and the world around them. We must understand this first in order to understand everything that follows within these pages.

It is certainly true that the practice of BDSM and various forms of kink can be considered non-normative. In 1992, anthropologist Gayle Rubin discussed what she described as the "Charmed Circle" of Western sexuality:

> Sexuality that is "good," "normal," and "natural" should ideally be heterosexual, marital, monogamous, reproductive, and non-commercial. It should be coupled, relational, within the same generation, and occur at home. It should not involve pornography, fetish objects, sex toys of any sort.
>
> Rubin, 2012

One of the most common micro-aggressions (or even simply aggressions) experienced by minority and marginalized communities is the pathologizing of their culture, practices, and relationships simply

DOI: 10.4324/9781003312833-1

because they fall outside of the mainstream. We know that this has commonly been the experience of BDSM practitioners, who disclose to mental or medical health providers that their sexual and relational identities fall outside of the Charmed Circle. This book seeks to offer a corrective to that experience.

That is why this is also a book about justice. Specifically, intimate justice and pleasure equity—terms coined by feminist academic Sara McClellan to capture the idea that all people are entitled to the experience of pleasure, as they each define it, and to critique the systemic barriers that prevent people from living authentic sexual and relational lives (McClelland, 2010). This book will introduce BDSM and kink to the reader from this perspective, understanding that kink stigma is a direct result of systemic reinforcement of the Charmed Circle idea of sexuality within healthcare and offering corrective knowledge from a culturally informed, kink-affirming perspective. This work begins with how we conceptualize our understanding of these terms.

WHAT WE MEAN WHEN WE TALK ABOUT "KINK"

At its core, "kink" is simply any sexual or relational practice that is non-normative for its place and time. These two qualifiers are crucial to our understanding of kink because what is considered kinky can and does change over time. In the Victorian era, masturbation was viewed as so horrifically maladaptive that parenting guides instructed young mothers to pin their children's nightgown sleeves to their bedding to prevent nocturnal self-touch (Oneill, 2019). While we like to think we have come a long way since one could mail order a barbed chastity device for one's teenager (Charleston, 2019), it was only 30 years ago, in 1994, that Surgeon General Joycelyn Elders was fired for suggesting that masturbation was a "part of human sexuality and . . . something that should be taught" in school sex education classes (Camacho, 2023). Today, the cultural conversation around self-pleasure has become more normalized. However, ideas around non-monogamy, power exchange, and sensory exploration within sexual play are still viewed with skepticism within both the medical and mainstream worlds.

This brings us to the other element contextualizing what "kink" means for us: the idea of place. While our understanding of "normal" sexuality (using the example of masturbation) has evolved over time, our conceptualization of what is "normal" depends not only on *when* we are having these conversations but *where*. A young man who opts out of traditional multi-husband "walking marriages" within the Mosuo people of China may be considered "kinky" by his local community, where matrilineal polyandry has been practiced since the 13th century (Johnson & Zhang, 1991). Likewise, homosexuality has been both legalized and (almost) entirely normalized within American society—but is still viewed as aberrant, socially harmful, and worthy of severe punishment in many parts of the world (Human Rights Watch, 2023). These variables are why it is crucial for anyone reflecting upon or attempting to assess a set of sexual or relational behaviors to be mindful of their own time and place—the cultural norms and values that may be informing their own understanding of what constitutes a "healthy" lifestyle.

This notion of Time+Place is reflected most explicitly in our conceptualization of fetishes and fetishistic desire: a sexual attraction toward an item or part of the body that is not typically understood as sexual. An understanding that genitals are sexual is relatively universal, and an erotic desire for or reaction to the penis and/or vulva is regarded as normative around the world. However, what is considered sexual or not varies depending (again) upon one's place and time. We can use bare breasts as our case in point. In places as disparate as the city parks of Berlin and the Koma tribal lands in Nigeria (Udodiong, 2019), toplessness—even full nudity—is normalized; whereas this is not the case in the United States. On the other hand, some places have seen their understanding of the sexualization of breasts change over time:

> Indonesian women didn't cover their breasts until Islam began to emerge there in the late 1200s. In India, toplessness was often a sign of class, depending on the region: Before Muslims entered north India in the 12th-16th centuries, only upper-class women covered their breasts; in the southwest region of Kerala, the majority ethnic group (Malayali) only allowed women of the Brahmin (priests and teachers) and Kshatriya (the ruling and military elite) castes to wear tops until 1858.
>
> Oyler, 2015

From the 16th to 18th centuries, visual erotica in the form of *Shunga* or "pillow books" were gifted to brides as a form of sex education in Japan. *Shunga* depicted group sex, female pleasure, homosexuality, and more in a style that emphasized joyful facial expressions and exaggerated genitals of all kinds (Artsy, 2013). On the other hand, in 21st century Japan—which still has a thriving erotica industry—the law requires that genitals be pixelated entirely (GQ India, 2017).

This erotic positioning within Time+Place extends beyond the body. In America, from colonial times through the mid-20th century, corporal punishment was the norm in most educational settings. The wooden paddle was seen as an educational implement to be wielded by parents and principals in order to discipline misbehaving children. This practice has dramatically declined over the last half-century, from 4% of children in 1978 to less than 0.5% in 2015; but it is still legal in 19 states today (Gershoff & Font, 2016). Perhaps in part due to this decline, the vast majority of Americans do not view paddles as educational or disciplinary objects. They have become wholly subsumed by their place within the world of BDSM impact play and are generally seen as entirely sexualized implements in a way that would not have been entirely appreciated 200 years ago. The cultural context of Time+Place extends throughout our understanding of fetishism and power play.

These cultural blind spots, when left unexamined, reinforce the "Charmed Circle" notion of Western sexuality, which then reaffirms hierarchies of vanilla over kink in turn and which results in what McKee et al. describe as a lack of interest in "whether the (behaviors) lead to consensual, happy sex that happens to be kinky . . . By doing so (they) exclude consent from discussions of healthy sex" (McKee et al., 2022). We cannot engage in productive dialog about any form of sexual, relational, or intimate expression without centering the concept of consent. In the words of Jemma Riedel-Johnson: "Consent is a proactive expression of what everyone is comfortable with instead of a reactive measure to what is already happening." When we center consent, we allow ourselves and each other not only the freedom to make choices that feel most comfortable for our own lives and relationships at the moment, but also the freedom to think critically about those choices and where they fall within the "Charmed Circle" our time and place afford.

SPEAKING OF WHICH . . .

This brings us to the topic of BDSM: a set of relational behaviors that have traditionally, and almost universally, been understood as existing outside the Charmed Circle of Western culture. BDSM is an acronym that contains three other acronyms nested within it:

- **BD**SM: Bondage and discipline.
- B**DS**M: Dominance and submission.
- BD**SM**: Sadism and masochism.

The following chapters will dive into each of these in depth. In short, bondage and discipline is best understood as an exchange of *control*: movement, speech, behavior, etc. It is commonly confused with dominance and submission: the exchange of *authority*. The best known of the three pairs is sadism and masochism (or sadomasochism), which we will define as an *exchange of sensation* for our purposes.

BDSM encompasses a broad spectrum of behaviors, practices, subcultures, and relationship styles that is impossible to fully expound upon in a single book. Thanks in large part to the power of modern technology and the ability of disparate people to connect with others who share similar interests and desires across large distances, the spectrum of intimate possibilities within the world of BDSM is expanding exponentially. It would be both impractical and unfair to suggest that a single introductory guide could offer a comprehensive picture of the full spectrum of BDSM expression. It is not inaccurate to say that this guide is, in some ways, already out of date.

While the body of academic work on BDSM and kink is still small (e.g., the American National Institutes of Health has yet to do a single study exploring alternative sexual expressions), the kink community itself is prolific. There are books, blogs, websites, and podcasts created for and about just about every possible iteration of BDSM/kink expression under the sun. Anyone seeking to understand the nature of BDSM expression must go beyond the world of peer-reviewed academic literature and engage with the work of BDSM practitioners themselves. The volume you now hold should be understood as a primer, offering a foundational roadmap toward the future study of the specific relationship models, sensory desires, or behavioral expressions you seek to understand. To this end, let us take a look at who and what we mean when we talk about "kinky" people and BDSM.

KINK DEMOGRAPHICS

It is challenging to study the demographics of the BDSM/kink community because, as for many other marginalized groups, historic stigma has led to a certain degree of healthy mistrust of those who would seek to classify and categorize its members. That said, a growing body of kink-identified and kink-affirming researchers have been working to study the world of BDSM in a way that is respectful, consent-based, and ethical.

Depending upon which research we consider, approximately 2–8% of the population identifies as kinky (De Neef, Huys, Morrens, & Coppens, 2019). BDSM and kink are more common within the LGBTQIA+ community (Richters et al., 2008); however, nearly 50% of individuals (across the spectrum of sexual orientations) surveyed acknowledge experimenting with BDSM (Holvoet et al., 2017); while 12.5% tell researchers that they engage in BDSM play regularly (De Neef et al., 2019). Among those who engage in BDSM play, a variety of motivators have been identified, including a view of kink as a cathartic escape from life (Baumeister, 1998); a form of "serious leisure"; and an expression of one's core erotic map (Sprott & Williams, 2019). Within the kink community, "evidence suggests that there are roughly equal proportions of dominants and submissives" (Connolly, 2006).

When exploring the origins of kinky desires, researchers have found that "43.4% of subjects describe their kink identity as being intrinsic . . . while 35.3% state that their interest was motivated by external influences" (Yost & Hunter, 2012). While one study exploring the origins of BDSM found that approximately one in five respondents connected their interest in kink to an originating trauma, this same study clarified that "most . . . who pointed to a traumatic event explained that their kink was an empowering way to cope with that event" (Hughes & Hammack, 2020). This is an important qualifier, since broader research has found that BDSM practitioners tend to report rates of trauma that are on par with the general population (Goerlich, 2020).

We know that kinky people ("kinksters") tend to be more educated than their vanilla peers and often hold white-collar, technical, or professional careers (ibid). While many studies report that approximately 80% of kinksters surveyed are white, we know that this is an ongoing sampling challenge that does not account for researchers' failure to seek out the spaces that BIPOC kinksters create for themselves and the cultural and safety considerations that lead study participants to self-select into or out of research. While not all kinky people are non-monogamous, we know that there is a healthy overlap between the BDSM and polyamory/ethical non-monogamy communities.

Finally, we know that—contrary to tropes and myths portraying kinky people as deviant or damaged—kinky people fall within the normal ranges for honesty-humility, empathy, emotionality, extroversion, agreeableness, conscientiousness, self-esteem, life satisfaction, and

Table 1.1 An Incomplete Taxonomy of Kink

	Sensation Players	Authority Exchange	Leather Folks	Bondage Players	Age Play	Pet Play	Gender Play	ENM
Femme Top		Domme Mistress Goddess	Leather Mommy		Mommy Nanny Governess			Cuckcake
Masc Top		Master Sir	Leather Daddy		Daddy Headmaster Teacher			Bull
Gender Inclusive Top	Sadist Sadomasochist Spanker Primal Predator	Dominant Disciplinarian Owner	Leather Top	Rope Top	Caregiver Big	Caregiver Handler Owner Trainer	Feminizer	Exhibitionist
Gender Inclusive Bottom	Masochist Spankee Primal Prey	Submissive slave property	Leather Bottom	Rope Bottom	ABDL Baby Babyboi Doll	Pet Puppy Pony Pig Hucow		Voyeur Toy
Femme Bottom		Brat Princess Kitten *Kajira*	Leathergirl	Rope Bunny (sometimes pejorative)	Babygirl Princess Kitten	Kitten	Sissy Doll Bimbo	Cuckquean

(*Continued*)

Table 1.1 (Continued)

	Sensation Players	Authority Exchange	Leather Folks	Bondage Players	Age Play	Pet Play	Gender Play	ENM
Masc Bottom		Kajirus	Leatherboy Leatherboi		Babyboy Prince			Cuckold
Femme Egalitarian			Leather-woman				Drag Queen	Cougar Hotwife Vixen
Masc Egalitarian			Leather-man				Drag King	Stag
Gender Neutral Egalitarian	Spanko Sensualist Hedonist		Bootblack	Rigger	Ageplayer	Fox		Swinger Hedonist Slut

desire for control. As one might expect, submissives scored higher than their Dominant peers in openness to new experiences and agreeableness; while Dominants were slightly more extroverted and desirous of control (Hébert & Weaver, 2014). We also know that BDSM practitioners are likely to have a stronger understanding of consent and be less likely to hold rape-supportive beliefs (Klement et al., 2017). In other words, by almost every metric available, researchers have found that BDSM practitioners are "just like everyone else," except for one minor difference: the way they form, structure, and express their sexual and intimate selves, alone and with their partners.

A BRIEF HISTORY OF KINK CULTURE

Fetishes have existed for as long as human beings have been manipulating materials to create new forms and tools. Dildos carved of ivory, rock, and bone have been found around the world—some dating back 28,000 years (Moskowitz, 2010). The oldest extant human figure found in the West is one of a pair of erotic figurines that copulate when joined together. Dubbed the "Adonis of Zschernitz," it dates back to 7200 BCE. It is particularly noteworthy since archaeologists suspect that the Adonis is not a fertility figure or deity, but rather likely our earliest example of pornographic art (Diver, 2005). The moment a new technology develops, humanity eroticizes it.

BDSM, on the other hand, is a slightly more nuanced conversation. For the vast majority of human history, the concept of consensual power exchange would have been incomprehensible. After all, as Janet Hardy and Dossie Easton observed in their classic work *The Bottoming Book*, power must first be *had* before it can be ceded to another (Hardy & Easton, 2001). For millennia, slavery was the global norm. Likewise, in most cultures worldwide, women were considered the chattels of their male relatives. The notion that one person could voluntarily give over their power to another would have been inconceivable—because the vast majority of people, in most places, across most of time, have never held personal power at all. While we can point to thousands of examples of sadomasochistic (giving and receiving intense sensation) behaviors in a myriad of cultures, these typically occurred either in a specifically religious context (e.g., the Roman Lupercalia) or as an "organic" element within cultures with a strict hierarchy of personhood. The idea that people could choose to enter into these dynamics or choose to step out of them did not exist because the autonomy necessary to enter into a power exchange relationship did not exist. To put it another way: consensual kink can only exist where equality is the social norm.

One of the earliest references to what could now be described as sexual masochism exists in the writings of a 17th-century medical text called *On the Use of Flogging in Venereal Affairs*. The author notes with satisfaction that "perverse cases" who derived erotic enjoyment of flogging would be "severely punished by avenging flames" (Meibom, 1650s). After all, self-mortification as an act of devotion to God (a common practice at the time) was holy; but the same act undertaken for self-pleasure was an affront. This practice emphasized the way that hierarchy (in this case, God and man) was understood also to regulate sexual desires. A century later, the Enlightenment and the new idea of equality among men would spark at least two revolutions—and a lot of randy behavior.

The Beggar's Bennison was a Scottish social group that counted some of the UK's elites among its members, who would gather to drink, carouse with sex workers, and engage in group masturbation on an elaborate silver platter (Stevenson, 2001). The Hellfire Club—founded by Sir Francis Dashwood—was equally ribald and often staged events that embraced both themes of the Pagan Bacchanalia and obscene parodies of Christian rituals, including sex workers dressed as nuns. Benjamin Franklin is believed to have been a frequent visitor during his time as an American ambassador in Europe (Goddard, 1972). These secret gentlemen's societies could only exist at a time when secular society was on the rise and the power of the church and state to regulate behaviors that would previously have been capital crimes had reduced the church's influence to mere social scandal.

As notions of human equality and suffrage spread around the globe, there was an increase in erotica that depicts what we might now call "power play." Pornographic postcards depicting chambermaids whipping their masters, for example, flourished in Europe after the invention of photography. The Reconstructionist era in the US gave rise to inexpensive erotic novels featuring interracial relationships, directly challenging the social and racial hierarchy of the day (Tupper, 2016). Moving into the 20th century, we see not only an increase in suffragist agitation but also a rise in pornography depicting powerful women dominating their male partners. There had to be an idea of equality before people could begin to play with (rather than live) paradigms of inequality.

Modern BDSM culture was deeply influenced by the experiences of gay military veterans returning home from World War II. Having already spent years together, many were unwilling to return to a closeted life back home in Middle America. They chose instead to remain in and around the cities where they were discharged from service: San Francisco for veterans of the Pacific Front, New York for those who served in Europe. These cities became thriving queer metropolises and their inhabitants looked to the past for examples of joyful same-sex relationships. Drawing from stories of romantic and erotic love in ancient Rome, Troy, and Sparta, this influenced the development of what we now know as Old Guard Leather and high-protocol Master/slave dynamics.

As the Queer Liberation movement grew in strength and force, lesbian women joined the community, with the first BDSM organization for women—Samois—being formed in 1978. They drew inspiration for their name from the city of Samois-sur-Seine, one of the settings featured in the classic BDSM novel *The Story of O*. The early 1980s and the rise of the AIDS crisis led to a new understanding of BDSM and kink: many longtime practitioners suggested that BDSM play could serve as a harm reduction strategy, allowing for deep connection, intimacy, and eros without the expectation of penetrative sex or the exchange of body fluids. These conversations coincided with the so-called Golden Age of Porn, when films such as *Deep Throat* and *Behind the Green Door* were played in mainstream movie theaters, inspiring a public conversation about sex, erotica, and kink that had never before occurred (McNair, 2012).

The 1980s took kink mainstream, with Anne Rice publishing (as A.N. Roquelaure) *Exit to Eden* and the *Sleeping Beauty Trilogy*—both of which depicted rich fantasy worlds of fetish play (spanking, specifically), sadomasochism, and domination and submission. Madonna embraced the same religious iconography that the Hellfire Club had eroticized 200 years earlier; and Hollywood churned out dozens of sexy thrillers that explored and exploited the power dynamics between their characters. By the early 2010s, kink had been mainstreamed by pop culture. The infamous *Fifty Shades of Grey* books had been published and suddenly everyone was talking about BDSM. Even with all of this, kinky people today still struggle to find positive representations of their lives and relationships. Fetishists in movies and on TV are still portrayed primarily as dangers to be avoided or "weirdos" to mock. Reality shows like *How to Build a Sex Room* pitch BDSM as a design esthetic as much as a path toward deeper relational connection. As we move through a time of social backlash toward gender, sexual, and erotic minorities such as queer and trans people, many kinksters are worried that they will be branded "groomers" or "deviants" by those who (much like the writer of *On the Use of Flogging in Venereal Affairs*) seek to impose their preferred social hierarchy by exerting control over the private lives of others. There is a vocal movement calling for the elimination of bodily autonomy for women and trans people—a rollback of laws that promote social equality, such as no-fault divorce and anti-discrimination provisions. Everything old is new again, but one thing remains the same: kink can only thrive in places and cultures where equality is the norm. We must have autonomy and agency outside of the bedroom before we can choose to cede it to our partners behind closed doors.

CULTURAL CONSIDERATIONS

It is a common misconception that BDSM/kink is a "white thing." This myth has been driven primarily by selection bias within studies of BDSM practitioners (Tatum & Niedermeyer, 2021). Erasure of BIPOC kinksters within both the academic literature and community content causes harm in the form of underrepresentation within research, microaggressions from both clinicians and other kinksters, and fetishization within the BDSM community.

> BDSM . . . is deeply informed by racialized sexual politics. Race is marginalized both within the scholarly literature and popular media about BDSM, contributing to the impression that it is not something black people do, should do, and/or that race is not a salient factor in the power dynamics so essential to the practice.
>
> Cruz, 2016

When clinicians fail to understand how BDSM/kink culture, practice, and language are understood and enacted by kinky clients from diverse racial and cultural backgrounds, they risk misunderstanding both the BDSM subculture and the unique framework with which their clients engage with kink.

One of the ways in which some BDSM practitioners engage with the intersection between race and culture and kink is through the notion of race play. "Race play" is the practice of negotiating and enacting scenes that center one or both partners' racial identities as core elements of the power exchange dynamic. This often takes the form of roleplay scenarios—such as a Nazi guard and a Jewish prisoner or an enslaved field worker and a plantation owner—that can be emotionally activating not only for the kinksters in the scene but for anyone else who happens to be observing.

> As a specific set of play practices, "race play" involves the intentional use of racial epithets or racist scenarios to help construct or maintain the exchange of power dynamics between participants. It is considered an edgier and even controversial practice by most BDSM practitioners because of the emotional labor and risk involved. Race play disallows the concealment of the presence of unequal racialized relations in BDSM practices precisely because it draws on real historical and contemporary relations of racism as a tool for constructing power dynamics.
>
> Oddie, 2022

Race play can be profoundly cathartic for the BIPOC kinkster who, thoughtfully and intentionally, uses BDSM as a tool to process intergenerational trauma, to reclaim their own sense of power and value, or to work through and recontextualize experiences of racism they have had in everyday life. However, all too often, the language and tropes of race play are co-opted by others who seek to act out their own racialized fetishes rather than genuinely engage with the deep work that race play can allow. Whether it is the Black man who is repeatedly asked to take on a bull roll within a cuckolding scene (a dynamic that plays into centuries of racialized fear of Black men); the Asian nonbinary individual who is assumed to be delicate, submissive, and eager to please; or the Jewish kinkster watching a stranger walk down a conference hallway wearing a leather Gestapo uniform, it is frustratingly common for minority kinksters to experience racism under the guise of race play. It is equally common and just as frustrating to be accused of "kink-shaming," being sex-negative, or being uptight/disconnected from themselves simply because they refuse to allow themselves to be objectified by others.

> Kink is not ONLY a cathartic tool. Just because someone is a member of a historically oppressed group or has a history of trauma does not mean that they want to use their kink expression to process these experiences. The fact that kink *can* be cathartic does not mean that kink *must be* cathartic. Sometimes people just want to have fun, and that's okay!
>
> Goerlich, 2023

Moving away from the specific practice of race play, the clinician must still be aware of the way the client's specific experience of culture (both their own and the dominant culture within which they live) informs and influences their understanding of BDSM/kink—specifically in their own understanding of power and control. For example, the language they choose to use may reflect their comfort levels with power exchange as a member of a religious, cultural, or ethnic minority group at both conscious and subconscious levels. One example of this is the use of the term "play" within the BDSM community to refer to the act of engaging in kink scenes. Someone who comes from a culture where playfulness is discouraged or looked down upon may embrace the idea of kinky play as yet another avenue for exploring the taboo of being naughty. It may be quite thrilling to "waste" their time playing at all, enhancing their psycho-sensory experience of the other scene elements. For others, the notion of play might bring up other emotions entirely and carry connotations that they find profoundly unsexy or unsettling.

> By defining play only through its pleasurable connotations, the term holds an epistemic bias towards people with access to the conditions of leisure . . . one that hurts as much as it heals and one that has been complicit in the systemic erasure of BIPOC people from the domain of leisure . . . We must urgently rethink the very definition of play so as to make space for those it has oppressed as well as those it has elevated.
>
> Trammell, 2020

The way our clients understand and connect to the notion of "play" and how their own cultural, religious, and racial identities are played with within kink spaces are just two examples of the importance of cultural competency within kink-affirming clinical practice. BDSM/ kink is not a "white thing"; however, the experiences of white kinksters have been centered and normalized as "the" kink experience for far too long. The kink-affirming clinician has an obligation not only to be informed of the specific language, rituals, practices, and ideas found within the BDSM subculture, but also to understand the culture of their client and the way that this informs the client's understanding of, connection to, and explorations of BDSM.

ADDITIONAL RESOURCES

The Ultimate Guide to Kink by Tristan Taormino
The Deep Psychology of BDSM and Kink by Douglas Thomas
Please Scream Quietly: A Story of Kink by Julie Fennell
Women and Kink: Relationships Reasons, and Stories by Jennifer Rehor and Julia Schiffman
The Color of Kink: Black Women, BDSM, and Pornography by Ariane Cruz

BONDAGE AND DISCIPLINE
Stefani Goerlich

THE EXCHANGE OF CONTROL

For some, "bondage" is the quintessential distillation of BDSM. When asked what constitutes "kink," their minds go straight to ropes and handcuffs (perhaps fuzzy), whips and chains. We will touch on whips in Chapter 4; but for now, let us explore what kinky people mean when they talk about "bondage" and its complementary kink, "discipline." What bondage and discipline have in common is that they are centered around the exchange of control. Bondage is the practice of exerting control over movement or speech—for example, through the use of restraints or gags. Discipline, on the other hand, is the control of behavior—such as through the introduction of writing lines, standing in the corner, restricting eye contact, or other forms of disciplined practice. While many think of corporal punishment—spanking, paddling, etc.—when they think of discipline, these behaviors actually represent an overlap between discipline and sadomasochism that is not necessarily present in every discipline dynamic. Bondage and discipline can be enacted within a relationship (e.g., when a Top ties their bottom to the bedframe) or solo (through the creation of self-imposed protocols, behaviors, and practices designed to evoke a power exchange dynamic). We will explore discipline in greater depth in the second half of this chapter.

DOI: 10.4324/9781003312833-2

BONDAGE

There is a reason that ropes and chains come to mind when one thinks of BDSM. Bondage is one of the most commonly reported sexual fantasies. In one study, 52% of women and 46% of men reported fantasizing about being tied up (Joyal et al., 2015). Twenty percent of study respondents tell researchers they have acted on these fantasies and brought restraints into their erotic play (Weisman, 2023). BDSM educator Jay Wiseman identifies three specific motivations/applications of erotic bondage:

- Bondage for vulnerability: "To restrict, in one way or another, their ability to move . . . if a person's ability to move is limited, then their ability to run away, fight off their 'attacker,' cover vulnerable parts of their body and so forth is also limited. In short, they are more vulnerable when they are bound than they are when they are not bound" (Wiseman, 2000).
- Bondage for decoration: This includes any kind of rope, restraint, or device applied to the person for the purpose of enhancing the aesthetics of their body or the moment. Decorative bondage can range from a collar around the neck (potentially signaling the relationship between Top and bottom) to a chastity device locked around the genitals; or an intricate *shibari*-style "beautiful ornamental body harness that's easy on the eyes and easier still on the body . . . not heavily constricting or physically challenging" (Midori, 2001) can be worn under the clothing comfortably all day, providing a gentle sensory reminder that the wearer is bound without needing to be visually obvious or overtly sexualized to achieve. Which brings us to Wiseman's third bondage application . . .
- Bondage for sensation: Bondage implements include a vast array of sensory and tactile options, ranging from abrasive ropes designed for discomfort to specialized restrictive clothing such as straitjackets and spools of common plastic wrap. Each of these evokes a specific sensory experience in the body of the wearer. A comforting, compression swaddle feels quite different than a suspended stress position—which means that parsing out the nuances of what "bondage" means for each person involved and negotiating which tactile sensations the soon-to-be-bound bottom would like to experience and which they would prefer to avoid are crucial elements of pre-scene negotiations.

Ropes and Restraints

The use of restraints within erotic encounters has a long history dating back to Ancient Greece and Rome. This is a broad category of tools that offers a spectrum of experiences catering to different preferences and comfort levels. While in some ways this represents the most simplistic form of bondage—often accomplished using basic household items and practiced by kinksters of wildly varying skill levels—there are several distinct forms of restraint play that we can identify:

- Sensory deprivation: We do not often consider the idea of sensory deprivation as a form of bondage, but understanding this bondage as the exchange of control (including controlling the amount of sensory input one experiences at any given time) helps us to contextualize this practice within the broader category of bondage and discipline. Sensory deprivation involves restricting one or more of the senses through the use of wearables such as blindfolds, hoods, gags, or earplugs. Limiting sensory input enhances the remaining sensations. For example, when one is blindfolded, the sense of touch heightens. When we are unable to hear, our vision tends to narrow and become more acute. Playing with enhancing or decreasing sensation can heighten arousal and intensify the overall experience for those involved.
- Bedroom bondage: An approach to bondage that often caters to beginners and those who prefer a more romantic/less intense power exchange experience, bedroom bondage often involves using texturally softer items—ranging from commercially made Velcro cuffs and sleep masks to repurposed everyday objects such as kitchen oven mitts and neckties—to affix oneself or one's partner to a bedpost, chair, or other furniture. The accessibility of these restraints, being freely available within the home or easily purchased from mainstream websites and mall stores, can feel less intimidating or overwhelming for folks who are curious about bondage and perhaps a bit wary about entering into "harder" BDSM spaces.
- Hard bondage: Hard bondage is characterized by the use of stronger, more restrictive, less yielding materials such as leather, chains, and other robust restraints. Unlike the softer materials of bedroom bondage, these are more likely to be buckled or locked into place rather than affixed with Velcro or ties, as many

bedroom bondage restraints are; and they may not be as easy to remove without help or cut through in an emergency. The choice of these heavier materials is central to the experience of hard bondage. Leather cuffs feel more substantial around the wrists and ankles than nylon restraints, and the weight of wearing chains can emphasize the feeling of surrender for those who wear them. Hard bondage implements afford a wide degree of creative possibility for BDSM practitioners. From "ballet boots" that limit the mobility of the wearer to the infinite flexibility of a length of chain and a handful of carabiner clips, these implements can range from the simplistic to the intricate and allow kinksters to customize and tailor the experience to their specific fantasies, sensory desires, and restriction preferences.

- *Shibari/kinbaku*: *Shibari* ("to tie" in Japanese) is a form of rope bondage that originated in Japan. Over time, *shibari* evolved from a practical martial art skill into a complex art form, emphasizing the beauty and symmetry of knots to create visually appealing patterns within a functional bondage restraint. While

Scan the QR Code above to see examples of decorative Shibari bondage. Warning: Some images contain nudity.

Figure 2.1   Decorative *Shibari* (QR code)

shibari emphasizes visual esthetics, *kinbaku* (or "tight binding") emphasizes the physical sensation of being restrained. As the name implies, *kinbaku* may involve intentional discomfort or pressure points, heightening the physical experience for the partner being bound. *Shibari* and *kinbaku* both utilize various types of knots, frictions, tensions, and hitches to create a wide range of patterns, designs, sensations, and degrees of restriction. *Shibari* and *kinbaku* go beyond the simple functionality of a hank of rope and emphasize the beauty, balance, and intentionality of the ties. Often practiced by skilled riggers who may have no other interest in BDSM, these skills are often embraced as art forms by practitioners rather than forms of alternative sexual expression.

- Self-bondage: As implied by the name, self-bondage is the practice of applying restraints to oneself for a variety of purposes. In some long-distance relationships, the submissive/bottom may engage in self-bondage at the direction of their Dominant as a form of connection and intimacy building. Additionally, folks who identify as "self-owned" may adopt certain bondage practices to reflect their status as such and to engage in aspects of power play, even in the absence of a partner. This allows them to experience an enjoyable "swing" between personal power and vulnerability. Self-bondage can take many forms, from simply wearing a subtle collar in daily life to more substantial restraints at home. Any form of bondage practiced alone requires meticulous planning, as the practitioner must be able to apply the restraint (which by definition will limit their senses or mobility to some degree) while also ensuring their physical safety and ability to self-release quickly. Because some forms of self-bondage (particularly when they involve the use of mechanical restraints such as cages or locks, as discussed below) carry a higher degree of risk, the use of "failsafe" mechanisms (e.g., ice locks) and safety planning are critical.

Mechanical Bondage

Mechanical bondage involves the use of specially crafted mechanical devices to secure, control, and restrict the movements of the individual being restrained. These can be static or motorized and are typically either fabricated out of materials like stainless steel, aluminum, and iron or created by modifying existing devices and machines. Unlike materials such as leather or rope, one of the appeals of mechanical bondage is the way that it can enhance the sensory experience of all partners in a scene by affording them opportunities to experience tactile sensations together, regardless of whether they are topping or bottoming in the scene. A classic example of this might be handcuffing. Both partners feel the sensation of cool metal against their warm skin as one partner places the handcuffs upon the other's wrists. Both feel the vibration of the cuffs ratcheting into place. Throughout the scene, both can hear the clink of metal against metal as the bottom moves their wrists. While only one partner is being restrained, they each experience multisensory stimuli that enhance their psychological experience and enjoyment of the scene. Another example is spreader bars—short metal bars with cuffs at either end used to keep the wearer's limbs apart and limit their ability to close their legs, use their hands, or walk easily. These emphasize the perception of vulnerability and exposure for the bottom and provide additional visual sensory input for the top.

Scan the QR code to see many examples of mechanical bondage by artist Jeff Gord during his life. Warning: Contains adult material. Please access with caution.

Figure 2.2 Mechanical Bondage (QR code)

Beyond these simple tools, more complex mechanical bondage devices have been developed by creative members of the BDSM community. Often integrated into predicament play scenes, these can include everything from lever and pulley systems to welded structures and retrofitted household and construction equipment to create intricate and highly customizable systems that allow users to exert precise control over the type, nature, and degree of restriction experienced by their partners. These creations highlight the ingenuity of many kinksters who adapt to the creative constraints of their local resources and develop playful new ways to control and have their movements controlled.

Not all mechanical devices are made of metal or involve the use of modern machines. Bondage enthusiasts often draw inspiration from the past as well. These iconic pieces of BDSM furniture are typically made of wood (although metal versions do exist), and their design is heavily influenced by historical accounts of devices used to punish transgressions against both church and state. The St. Andrews Cross is a large X-shaped standing structure with attachment points at each corner for the wrists and ankles to hold the person being restrained in a position that spreads their limbs wide, leaving the entirety of their exposed body free for whatever they and their Top have planned. The St. Andrew's Cross has come to be seen as both a simple, practical restraint and a symbol of submission within BDSM. A stockade is more complicated to fabricate but has grown in popularity in both erotica and real-life usage. Also called "stocks," a stockade is typically either freestanding or placed around the neck of the bottom, confining their head and hands. Someone placed in stocks may find themselves kneeling, standing, or bent at the waist, unable to move their head or arms, intensifying their feelings of "helplessness" and exposure. The inherent simplicity of the St. Andrew's Cross and the stockade adds to their popularity and effectiveness. Overall, mechanical bondage introduces a unique dimension to BDSM practices, which can be shared in some sense by all involved in the scene. From the cold touch of metal devices and the rough texture of wooden restraints to the intricate designs of advanced machines, both fantastical and practical, mechanical bondage allows practitioners to explore new realms of pleasure, vulnerability, and power together.

Predicament Play

Predicament play can serve as a connective thread between bondage and discipline because it is predicated both on the positioning and limitations imposed upon the bottom and on the decisions they make around how to adapt to these limitations. Predicament play often takes the form of "forced choice" scenarios that require the submissive to navigate multiple emotional needs and/or sensory experiences. The element of choice/ambiguity on the part of the partner placed into the predicament situation adds a mental/ emotional element to the scene that can heighten both the physical sensation experienced by the submissive and the energetic dynamic between themselves and their top.

The most classic forms of predicament play involve the bottoming partner holding a specific position (e.g., standing on tiptoes) for prolonged periods of time. Failure to maintain the posture results in the administration of some form of sensation—for example, contact with a powerful vibrator when the submissive lowers their feet or the pull of a rope (that is loose as long as the wearer remains on tiptoes). The predicament here is the submissive's self-discipline in holding the mandated position, even as fatigue sets in and it becomes physically uncomfortable, versus choosing to adjust their position and thereby accept the (perhaps unpleasant) consequences. The process of navigating the predicament they find themselves in—balancing their physical needs and limits against their mental fortitude and emotional desire to serve and please—is often the most intense and pleasurable part of the predicament play experience for the submissive.

This mental element is where discipline comes into the scene:

> When you restrain someone with rope or other tools, you're taking (many of) their choices away. But if you simply tell someone to hold still, they're doing it because you said so, and because they want to please you—that's powerful stuff. Something as brutally simple as putting a sticker or drawing a circle on a wall and telling your submissive to put their nose on the sticker/drawn circle and not move, under pain of earning your disappointment, is quite the predicament . . . That's where the real power of this kind of play lies. The only thing keeping them in that position is the mental desire to obey and please the person that gave them the command.

> Harris, 2023

DISCIPLINE

It is a common misconception that when kinky people talk about "discipline," they are referring to physical discipline, such as spanking. While that certainly can be a part of many power exchange dynamics, in BDSM, "discipline" refers to something much deeper and often much less physical.

When thinking about the concept of discipline within the context of control exchange, the goal is to consider the mental processes of self-discipline and obedience. Often, in BDSM relationships, this takes the form of cultivating and following negotiated rules, rituals, and protocols. These are distinct yet interconnected concepts that govern behavior, communication, and interactions within various contexts—including the workplace, the family hierarchy, and kinky and vanilla interpersonal relationships. While each serves different purposes, they share some commonalities and often overlap in practice. The following paragraphs will delve into the differences and similarities between rules, rituals, and protocols.

Rules

Rules are the expectations for specific actions or behaviors that are codified and agreed upon by the members of a particular system, organization, or society. Rules are typically explicit, enforceable, and designed to uphold the standards and expectations of those creating them. Well-created rules are clear and specific, leaving little room for misunderstanding or misinterpretation. They define the parameters of what is allowed or prohibited within the organization, group, family, or dyad. Traffic laws are an excellent example of social rules: the white and yellow lines painted on the road are not barricades. They are easily crossable. And yet each driver forms an agreement with their fellow drivers to obey the traffic rules they represent. When these rules of the road are violated, there can be consequences—both "natural" (damage to the car) and social (a ticket). Rules carry with them an implicit understanding that corresponding penalties or consequences are possible when violated. Legal statutes, corporate guidelines, social media user agreements, and power exchange contracts have defined behavioral expectations (rules) and associated punishments for those who break them. Rules are a form of authority exchange existing in every setting and society, whether the agreements are formed intentionally or entered without conscious decision.

Establishing clear rules within our relationships has multiple benefits for everyone involved. We can define our personal boundaries and set clear expectations for ourselves and those around us. This can include everything from how we wish to communicate with one another, our expectations for personal space, and how we prefer to give and receive feedback and navigate conflict resolution. When everyone has clarity around the rules for a given relationship, understands them, and mutually agrees to abide by them, it goes a long way to preventing misunderstandings and resolving conflicts before they spiral out of control. In power exchange dynamics, rules may include agreements on how to address disagreement between the partners in a way that allows each to feel heard without needing to step out of their dynamic or feel as if they are failing to live up to the expectation of being a "good" Dominant/submissive/etc. In all relationships, but perhaps especially in power exchange relationships, rules can create a sense of predictability, constancy, and trust. When we know what to expect from each other, we feel more secure and trust can build over time.

Rituals

Rituals are specific actions, routines, or ceremonies that hold cultural, social, or personal significance. They often follow specific patterns or routines and spotlight important events, transitions, or meaningful moments. Rituals are rich in symbolism and shared meaning, and can be religious (Catholic high mass), nationalistic (Fourth of July fireworks displays), familial (unique Thanksgiving traditions), and social (sorority initiations) in nature. Rituals are deeply ingrained aspects of all human societies. They can range from small daily practices (making an offering to Hotei before opening a restaurant each day) to marking significant life milestones such as child-naming ceremonies and funerals. These ritual moments often feature specific gestures that can be simple and are often familiar across cultures—lighting two candles on Shabbat or blowing out candles on a birthday cake, for example—but the recitation of specific, formalized words or the addition of meaningful movements and gestures creates a psychological impact that goes far deeper than the behavior itself might indicate to outside observers. The repetition of these ritualized words, gestures, and moments reinforces their significance and serves as a way to connect people and groups across time and geography. Cultural rituals (including those of the BDSM subculture) and adherence to social norms provide a sense of continuity, belonging, and meaning. Particularly for folks experiencing isolation from their community or culture, adopting an individual ritual practice can help foster a sense of identity and purpose that can be an important resilience factor, helping them navigate both significant milestones and challenges.

Power exchange rituals are a way for kink-identified individuals or partners in power exchange relationships to reinforce their roles, deepen their connection, and create a sense of structure and intimacy within their dynamic. These predictable, meaningful moments and actions serve to cultivate, maintain, and enhance the bond between partners. Rituals serve to honor and acknowledge the importance of both small daily gestures and significant milestones in a relationship—such as a submissive returning their collar to his Dominant following a breakup. Acknowledging these moments through ritual reinforces the importance of the experience for all involved. Rituals can serve as a source of comfort and acknowledgment in good times and bad. Examples of power exchange rituals could include the following:

- **Journaling**: Many Dominants ask their submissives to keep a journal documenting their feelings, experiences, and thoughts related to their lives, their mental health, their submission, and more. This is both a personal growth and mindfulness practice and a way of communicating with one another. In many power exchange relationships, the submissive's journal entries may be read by their Dominant as a way both to offer insights into the submissive's headspace and to deepen the emotional and communicative bond between them.
- **Morning or evening rituals**: Consistent rituals to mark the start or end of each day can be a powerful connective force within the power exchange relationship. Whether this takes the form of a submissive kneeling by the Dominant's bedside each morning to greet them or the Dominant brushing their submissive's hair each evening before bed, both partners can adopt small connective practices that add deep meaning to the day and tenderness to the relationship.
- **Task-based rituals**: Service-oriented rituals involve the bottoming or submissive partner performing specific tasks to please their Top and make their day more manageable and pleasant. Tasks such as preparing breakfast in bed each morning, making

sure the bills are paid each month, or offering a massage at the end of the day can be a lovely way to reinforce and externalize the power exchange dynamic.

- **Punishment rituals**: When a submissive fails to obey a rule or complete an assigned task, discipline is often the expected outcome. When punishment is ritualized, the gravity of this breach is emphasized in the minds of both the authority holder and the one who serves them. Punishment rituals may include the bottoming partner selecting the implement that will deliver the punishment, reserving a specific place, tool, or position for negative reinforcement exclusively; or the use of humiliation/degradation to reinforce behavioral expectations.

- **Collaring/consideration ceremonies**: For many within the kink community, a collaring ceremony is a significant ritual—in some cases akin to, or even more meaningful than, a wedding ceremony, and sometimes just as public. During a collaring ceremony, the Dominant places a collar (ranging in type from a leather buckled collar to a solid metal ring to a delicate jeweled necklace) on their submissive as a symbol of ownership, commitment, and submission. Often, the submissive will kneel or bow as the collar is placed around their neck, signifying their dedication to the Dominant. Vows of some kind may be exchanged or a contract signed. Often, for kinky couples, the collaring ceremony is woven into their legal wedding ceremony. In some hierarchical forms of BDSM, there may be an intermediate step before a formal collaring, known as being taken under consideration or protection. These are often public declarations that the submissive has chosen to offer some degree of deference to the Dominant but that either they also retain some "free agency" or the power exchange relationship is not yet a permanent one.

Because the creation and implementation of ritual is a universal norm, it is possible for ritualized behaviors that would exist within power exchange dynamics to be adopted by individuals without partners ("self-owned submissives"). Likewise, rituals may carry over and replicate from one relationship to the next without significant alteration from partner to partner. It is important to be mindful that because so much of our cultural practice is expressed through ritualized behavior, there is always a risk of ritualized behavior being adopted unconsciously or without much explicit negotiation. When working with or entering into power exchange dynamics, we need to be clear that all rituals are being negotiated, consented to, and adapted to suit the needs and preferences of all parties in the relationship. Communication, trust, and mutual respect are vital elements in developing and implementing power exchange rituals. Of course, all activities within a BDSM or power exchange dynamic should prioritize the safety and wellbeing of all parties involved.

Protocols

A "protocol" is a "code prescribing strict adherence to correct etiquette and precedence" (Merriam-Webster, 2023) in a given hierarchical (e.g., military) or cultural context. Protocols are less stringent than rules and are typically understood as a set of best practices or expected conventions within a given people-group, place, or time. Protocols are adaptable to different situations and can be adjusted as needed, even as they represent the "ideal" set of behaviors and responses to any given circumstance or situation. Protocols are best understood as a general framework rather than strict directives. In many settings, adherence to the protocol is voluntary and predicated on cultural understanding and mutual cooperation among participants. For example, it is an expected protocol at many kink events that one does not approach or speak to a submissive without first asking their Dominant if they may do so. Doing so when the submissive is not attending solo would be considered a serious breach of etiquette. This is one example of how communities and organizations develop conventions, customs, and best practices that enhance the experience for everyone within that particular context. Ideally, protocols serve as cultural reference points for efficient, effective, and respectful interactions.

When protocols are established within power exchange relationships, they are used to define the dynamic and emphasize the roles of topping and bottoming partners. The relationship protocols within a BDSM relationship can vary widely based on personal preferences and the nature of the relationship. In many power exchange dynamics (both long and short term), it is common for participants to create protocols such as the following:

- **Greetings and farewells:** The submissive may be required to greet the Dominant in a specific manner, such as by kneeling, when they meet or enter a room. Likewise, there may be a departure protocol, such as asking for permission before leaving the Dominant's presence.

- **Wardrobe:** The authority holder may dictate what their bottoming partner wears either on a daily basis (even outside of BDSM activities) or on specific days or occasions to reinforce their control and establish a particular esthetic. This can range from specific nail polish colors or hairstyles to requiring the submissive to wear specific lingerie, collars, or other accessories.
- **Use of honorifics:** Protocols for how the submissive addresses the Dominant might include using honorifics like "Sir/Ma'am," "Lady," "Daddy," or any other terms of endearment. Likewise, a submissive might be referred to as "girl/boy," "little one," "princess," or "pig," to name just a few of the many appellations available.
- **Service expectations:** Specific tasks or duties may be carried out regularly in a structured way that align with the submissive's role and emphasize the nature of the power dynamic—such as serving meals in a specific way, laying out clothing on a daily basis, or engaging in acts of anticipatory service—where the goal is to meet the Dominant's need before it is even voiced.
- **Punishments and rewards:** Mutually agreed upon systems can reward obedience to negotiated rules, compliance with established rituals, and an ongoing habit of good behavior—however that is defined within the dynamic. This may be tracked using tools such as sticker charts or task-sharing apps and often involves the dispensing of praise, privileges, or special treats. Alternatively, when rules are broken and rituals or protocols fall by the wayside, the authority-holding partner may choose to punish the mutually defined poor behavior (see the following section).

As in all things related to consensual power exchange, protocols should be negotiated by both the Dominant and submissive rather than unilaterally prescribed. Regular communication, trust, and the ability to renegotiate, adapt, and modify protocols as needed for the wellbeing, safety, and pleasure of everyone involved are essential to maintaining a healthy power exchange relationship.

A negotiated combination of rules, rituals, and protocols can create a relationship framework that promotes healthy attachment, clear boundaries, and general happiness for all involved. For example, establishing rules for clear communication can prevent misunderstandings that can lead to unearned punishment or unnecessary frustrations; while having rituals for emotional connection (e.g., dedicated date nights) and celebrating milestones (e.g., collaring ceremonies or annual contract renegotiation) can help to nurture and sustain the emotional bond. Protocols for addressing conflict within the power dynamic can ensure that disagreements are resolved respectfully and constructively. None of these practices is a relationship panacea. The efficacy of rules, rituals, and protocols in relationships depends on the mutual agreement and adoption by all partners (rather than the unilateral imposition by one on the other) and a willingness to adapt them as necessary as the relationship evolves. When used thoughtfully and in a way that prioritizes the wellbeing of both parties, rules, rituals, and protocols can contribute to healthier, more fulfilling interpersonal relationships—both kinky and vanilla.

Punishments

The idea of punishment existing within an interpersonal or romantic/marital relationship is one that gives many people pause. Obviously, within non-hierarchical or egalitarian relationship structures, punishment plays no role and can be seen as an indicator of intimate partner violence. While it is quite possible to have a mutually satisfying power exchange relationship that does not involve the infliction of punishment by one partner to another within authority and/or control exchange relationships, some form of consequence for failure to adhere to the negotiated power exchange agreements is expected. Punishments vary widely, depending upon the specific nuances and desires of each power exchange partnership, but often include one or more of the following:

- **Time out/solitude:** Standing in a corner; sitting separately; speech restrictions.
- **Loss of privileges:** No television or video games; reduction/ elimination of favorite activities; revocation of progress on goal/ sticker charts.
- **Extra tasks:** Household chores; large projects such as detailing a car; "timewaster tasks" such as sorting colored beads or counting grains of rice.
- **Loss of socialization:** Skipping a play party; staying home while their partner attends a munch.
- **Sleep changes:** Going to bed earlier than usual; sleeping separately; sleeping on the floor.

- **Formal apology:** The implementation of an apology protocol, which may include specific postures/positions, lowered head/eyes, and specific word expectations.
- **Writing lines or essays:** Writing sentences such as, "I will not touch the vibrators while my Sir is at work" 200 times or writing a 500-word essay explaining what happened, why, and what lesson can be learned from the situation.
- **No dessert:** Access to healthy foods or water should never be restricted as a form of punishment. However, denial of desserts, sweets, or alcoholic beverages may be appropriate.
- **Taking away toys/devices:** Denial of a favorite sex toy or impact tool; being temporarily uncollared or switched to a less favored collar; for age players, removal of actual stuffed animals, toys, coloring books, etc. (Note that removal of a collar—even temporarily—can be an incredibly serious consequence for misbehavior and could be construed as a comment on the stability/longevity of the relationship.)
- **Somatic punishments:** Spanking; a specific number of strikes with a disfavored impact tool; orgasm denial; holding specific poses for a set length of time; chastity.

As we acknowledge the aforementioned discomfort that comes when mainstream, aiming-for-egalitarian relationship culture considers negotiated power exchange dynamics, we must also consider the fact that, for those in hierarchical relationships, punishment can serve to reinforce positives within the relationship. These may include the following:

- **Responsibility:** Punishments that enforce the responsibilities of the partners can be a tool for rebuilding trust and reconfirming consent. Understanding the division of authority within a kink dynamic is necessary for all parties to be able to offer ongoing consent and to understand what the boundaries of the relationship agreement are, since it is not uncommon for rule violations to represent a subtle resistance to, or objection to, the existing power exchange paradigm. A formalized process for responsibility-taking can also become a pathway toward renegotiating the relationship agreement.
- **Boundaries:** As mentioned above, when boundaries are violated in any context, a mechanism for repairing that relationship

breach is necessary. Punishment can be a useful tool of restoration in these moments—particularly punishments that provide an opportunity for one person to constructively do something for the other, such as a ritual moment, a task, or a letter.

- **Accountability:** Power exchange of any form, even in dynamics that do not include authority exchange, is predicated on a high degree of trust. The ability to know that the person wrapping you in ropes or running the flat of a knife down your back should be one you can scrupulously rely on to honor their word and fulfill their obligations. It is essential to have a mechanism to hold each other accountable and to recognize when a simple mistake or an egregious violation has occurred. Accountability punishments are common within community spaces when someone fails to follow the rules of a given event or venue and can be written into relationship agreements to afford the submissive partner a process to address grievances with their Dominant without stepping outside of their dynamic to do so.

- **Behavior modification:** Some of the most common rules created within kinky relationships are those related to self-care and healthy behaviors: rules about taking daily prescriptions, drinking adequate water, or participating in routine exercise are all fairly standard. Punishments can serve as incentives to implement new behaviors and eliminate harmful habits (e.g., smoking) from one's daily routine. Behavior modification is entirely possible without the external motivator of power exchange; but having that extra incentive that BDSM affords, or the ability to "eroticize" a necessary but uncomfortable lifestyle change, can be a boon to many kinky people.

- **Safety:** Nothing is intrinsically safe. Every behavior has an element of risk, from watching television on the couch to running an ultra-marathon. Within BDSM, an ongoing awareness of safety best practices is necessary in every context, scene, and relationship dynamic. When safety protocols are violated, punishments such as ejection from a group or community, loss of access to a particular toy or piece of equipment, or even the end of a relationship are the norm.

- **Reinforcing authority:** BDSM is a hierarchical form of connection. Some hierarchies last a few moments ("You have the power to inflict sensation upon me for the duration of our wax play scene, but I am not going to listen to your demands after we end the scene"); while others endure for decades ("I will be your owned pet for the rest of our lives and obey your every directive"). For the most part, those involved in power exchange dynamics find comfort in a clearly defined hierarchy. There are dynamics that play with hierarchy, such as "bratting"—where the bottoming partner playfully resists or subverts their top's will in order to evoke reactions and "punishments" from them. Whether playful bratting or a more stressful imbalance between the partners, punishment can be one way of restoring the hierarchical equilibrium.

- **Consistency:** Whether the context is modifying behavior, reinforcing the partnership dynamic, or ritualizing the process of repair after a relationship breach, having a consistent and predictable way to enact these moments can help build and maintain healthy attachments and stronger bonds between the partners. Much like the parent-child relationship, the ability to anticipate outcomes and trust that those we love will respond to us in consistent, trustable ways is also a core need in adult relationships—particularly for those with chosen hierarchy and self-selected power imbalances.

- **Resolving conflict:** Conflict is an inevitable part of every relationship and is not a bad thing in and of itself. Conflict is how we grow as individuals and managing conflict is a key emotional intelligence skill. Punishments can serve as a vehicle for reparation and atonement for both partners. Having a physical outlet for emotional hurt (through sadomasochistic play) or a ritualized or structured way to express our remorse, co-created, negotiated punishment can be a tool of healing for folks in power exchange dynamics.

We cannot end this section without emphasizing that punishment within any relationship or partner group should be mutually agreed upon, balanced, and constructive. Punishments that "outweigh the crime" or that are experienced as coercive can have negative consequences, such as damaging power-exchange relationships, causing emotional harm (to one or more partners), and even drifting into the realm of abuse. The spectrum of punishments possible within a kinky dynamic should always be determined well ahead of any potential behavioral breach, negotiated by all involved, and consistent from incident to incident and partner to partner. Choice and agency are always present within a healthy power exchange. As such, punishments should not be imposed by the dominant partner so much as conceded to or undertaken by the submissive.

SAFETY AND RISK

As with all physical activities, from jumping on a trampoline to jogging in the park, bondage and discipline carry certain elements of risk. While this is more common for the former than the latter, an important element of providing kink-affirming psychoeducation is having an awareness of red (or yellow) flags so that we may support our clients in avoiding harm where possible. It is important to note that the ultimate authority on what is harmful to the client should be the client themselves. The clinician is there to ask motivational questions, to help the client identify their strengths, and to support them in developing their own personal risk framework—which will often vary from that which the clinician would have for themselves. It is never the job of the clinician to tell the client what they "should" or "should not" do; but rather to guide the process of self-reflection, boundary setting, and risk tolerance reflection so that the client can ultimately decide for themselves (free from the influence of either practitioner or partner) what they feel most comfortable doing or not.

With this caveat in mind, there are some practices that should raise concern for the kink-affirming clinician and indicate that a safety planning conversation with the client is warranted. These include the following:

- **Self-bondage or auto-erotic bondage:** While there are many skilled bondage practitioners who can self-tie without needing the extra pair of hands a partner can provide, it is generally accepted that bondage play while alone carries a degree of risk that is best avoided. Any number of circumstances may arise—ranging from an overly tightened knot to a full-blown medical emergency—that are best addressed by another (unbound) person. Additionally, mechanical bondage used to enhance the effects of orgasm, a practice commonly referred to as "autoerotic asphyxiation," can cause severe injury or even death in a matter of moments. "The estimated annual incidence of sexual asphyxia is 2–4 cases per million in the United States . . . The most common mechanism of autoerotic death is by ligature asphyxiation. Experimentation with other methods such as plastic bag asphyxia, inhalation of noxious chemicals, aqua-eroticum (autoerotic drowning), and electricity have resulted in a fatality while striving for sexual gratification" (Shields & Hunsaker, 2020). Mechanical bondage for autoerotic pleasure, whether practiced alone or with a partner, has a high degree of lethality and should be explored with the client upon disclosure.

- **Bondage under the influence:** Alcohol, the most commonly used intoxicating substance (Prottle, 2023), has been linked in hundreds of studies to poor decision-making and perceptual reasoning. Alcohol intoxication impairs attention, "enhancing an individual's focus on the most salient, easy-to-process cues, limiting the ability to attend simultaneously to competing cues that would inhibit problematic behavior" (Davis-Stober et al., 2019). It is no surprise, then, that someone engaging in bondage while intoxicated may struggle to monitor their partner's verbal cues, the color and temperature of their extremities, the skill of their knotwork, and their own wakeful alertness simultaneously. Unfortunately, failing to take repeated note of each of these variables increases the risk of injury during a scene. If this is true for something as "harmless" as a glass or two of wine before a scene, how much greater is the danger when illicit substances are added to the equation? As Wiseman puts it: "It has been very obvious to me that intoxicant use was an 'essential co-factor' in many SM-related disasters, and that had intoxicant not been used it is quite possible that the incident would never have happened . . . I have concluded that intoxicant use by any person in the scene automatically increases the degree of risk . . . and that intoxicant use by both people automatically takes the scene up to the 'extreme' degree of risk" (Wiseman, 2000).

- **Pain or numbness during bondage play:** Obviously, there is an expectation of sensation that comes with engaging in bondage play and, to a lesser extent, discipline (e.g., kneeling on grains of rice; writing lines). These sensations can sometimes be purposefully unpleasant, but there is a distinction to be made between acceptable sensation and sensation that raises safety concerns for the participants. "Disruption of circulation is the primary safety concern related to . . . bondage. This is because lack of circulation in any part of the body, regardless of whether it occurs in a region of a major artery or capillary network, can lead to tissue damage—including bruising, temporary or permanent nerve damage, and in extreme, unmitigated situations, necrosis (tissue death)" (Dan & JD, 2009). While we often think of these risks being most common with rope bondage, other restraints such as overly tightened cuffs, zip ties, and mechanical bondage devices, as well as stress positions or prolonged time holding a specific body posture, can also have deleterious effects on the body.

- **Using unsafe or untested equipment:** Riggers, or those who identify primarily as bondage practitioners, are not dissimilar to the wine sommelier—trained in the subtle differences between various materials and how each can enhance or hinder the overall experience of the whole. From coconut fiber rope and smithed steel to 3D printing and strongly worded commands, bondage practitioners can elucidate the precise ways each material will act on the body when handled with care and skill. Like wine, there are a variety of factors that blend together to create a safe and enjoyable bondage scene. These range from a working knowledge of anatomy and first aid to understanding which materials can be safely used to restrain a partner and which should be avoided. It is the latter factor that can cause problems for some whose enthusiasm outpaces their formal knowledge of BDSM.

- **Lack of skill-building education:** It is NOT the clinician's role to take on the task of educating clients about safe BDSM practices. However, a kink-affirming provider should be well versed in the body of available educational resources in order to point their client toward appropriate skill-building material. Additionally, it is both ethical and appropriate to ask questions about a client's bondage practice—expressing curiosity about their equipment safety protocols in the same way we might if we discovered that they were avid skydivers. Motivational interviewing combined with psychoeducation about how to access kink-affirming education should be an element of any kink-affirming clinician's risk assessment and safety planning process.

ADDITIONAL RESOURCES

Jay Wiseman's Erotic Bondage Handbook by Jay Wiseman

The Sensual Art of Japanese Bondage by Midori

The Ultimate Guide to Bondage: Creating Intimacy through the Art of Restraint by Mistress Couple

Better Bondage for Every Body: With Rope Bondage Experts From Around the World by Evie Vane

Somatics for Rope Bottoms: 12 Embodied Inquiries for Transforming Your Experience in Rope Bondage by Natasha NawaTaNeko

DOMINANCE AND SUBMISSION
Elyssa Helfer

AUTHORITY EXCHANGE

Making decisions, giving orders, and enforcing obedience: in the non-kink world, these concepts—derived from the *Oxford Languages* definition of "authority"—are not particularly sexy (Oxford Dictionary). Whether coming from bosses, parental figures, teachers, law enforcement officers, or politicians, we would be hard pressed to find someone in a position of power who is not asserting (or attempting to assert) their authority over us. Power hierarchies are deeply embedded within our current systems, whether or not we are consenting to or consciously aware of our participation in them. In various realms of our lives, we cannot escape authority; but authority is precisely what is sought in one particular realm. As its name suggests, the consensual exchange of authority is a fundamental thread that permeates the relational dynamics of dominance and submission (D/s). In some cases, this exchange takes place in particular contexts, negotiated to exist only during a pre-negotiated time or within a particular space. For others, the exchange of authority is permanent and encompasses all aspects of the lives of those participating. As with all kink-related interactions, informed consent is a prerequisite for participation within an authority exchange dynamic and negotiation of the terms of the dynamic should be ongoing; what works for a relationship today may be different than what works for that relationship tomorrow.

Within the kink community and among kink-specializing academics, researchers, and clinicians, the terms "power exchange,"

DOI: 10.4324/9781003312833-3

"authority transfer," and "authority exchange" have all been utilized to describe the hierarchical dynamics that exist when one
person yields their power to another. Whether debating in a class-
room setting or in a Reddit thread, the question continues to arise:
which of these terms is correct? As it will become clear (if it has not
already), kink dynamics are highly personal, fluid, and expansive. The
debate over which term is correct will likely not conclude as a new
term will emerge once a consensus is reached, and the process will
begin again. So, while we can sit within the ever-growing and likely
never-ending debate, I invite you to lean into what resonates most
strongly with you; and if that happens to be something aside from
what is used in this chapter, please note that I am not the foremost
"authority" (see what I did there?) on how you do, will, or should
define your particular dynamic. That said, for the purpose of consistency, this chapter will utilize the term "authority exchange."

Within an authority exchange dynamic, kinky folks typically fall
into one of three roles. The first is the role of the "Dominant." The
person who takes on the dominant role may not necessarily define
themselves as a "Dominant" (there are a variety of dominant personalities, which will be expanded upon below); however, they are
in the position of power within the dynamic, asserting their control
over whoever is yielding their power. The type of control that they
assert will depend on the negotiated dynamic; however, what remains
consistent within the "dominant" subgroup of kinksters is that they
are in a *consensual pre-negotiated* position of power. The person who
relinquishes their power is the "submissive." Again, the person who
undertakes the submissive role may not necessarily refer to themselves as a "submissive"; instead, they may identify more strongly with
another identity that takes on a submissive role. However, submissives
consensually position themselves lower within the power hierarchy.
Lastly, a "switch" is someone who identifies with both dominance and submission and whose fluidity between those roles shifts
depending on the relational, social, or sexual circumstances.

A common discourse within the kink community is whether the
Dominant truly holds the power when the submissive has a say—
based on the consensual negotiation—about what the kink dynamic
will look like and holds the power to revoke consent at any time.
Thus, is the submissive really the one with all the power? You will
likely hear different answers each time you ask this question, as the
individual experiences of those within these dynamics will differ

based on a variety of factors. Author Emma Turley (2018) notes that "power exchange is multilayered, and therefore dominant and submissive partners have equal responsibilities and influence during BDSM, though these are enacted in different ways." Staci Newmahr, however, notes that it is the importance of *belief* in the agency of the submissive/bottom that allows for the hierarchy to feel authentic:

> This belief in SM [sadomasochism] as the actual transfer of control hinges on the suspension of belief in the agency of the bottom. At its core, the link between SM participants is a quest for a sense of authenticity in experiences of power imbalance. To achieve this, participants must suspend belief in their own egalitarian relations for the duration of the scene. When this is successful, the sense of power imbalance feels real. This is sought, and what often occurs, in and through power exchange. SM participants seek authenticity in emotional, physical, and psychological experience, rather than authenticity in their presentation to others. I use "authenticity" to refer to participants' feelings and experiences of relative powerfulness or powerlessness, during and as a consequence of their SM scenes. This achievement of authenticity is beyond that of what one might experience when playing a role. In other words, SM participants who, when they play, feel as if they are playing a role (as an actor might) do not achieve the authenticity of players who say that they feel afraid, helpless, evil, or invincible during their play. Unlike in improv or other kinds of performance, the authenticity in SM lies in the extent to which SM participants are able to convince themselves, and each other, of the realness of the experience.
>
> Newmarh, 2010

Whether for a scene or a lifetime, authority exchange dynamics are grounded in consent, mutual desire, and, of course, pleasure—which certainly makes decision-making, giving orders, and enforcing obedience a whole lot more appealing.

TOTAL POWER EXCHANGE

In addition to consent, another essential aspect of healthy kink engagement is effective, thorough, and honest communication. This is particularly important as kinky folks delve deeper into the dynamics within the BDSM community that are inherently riskier.

> Emphasizing communication should lead to a better understanding among participants regarding individuals' unique identities, needs, and motivations, and thus more fulfilling BDSM experiences. In short,

communication as its own entity allows for participants to better understand the subjective realities of those with whom they play.

Williams et al, 2014

To be clear, communication should be emphasized in *all* kink engagement; however, it is of paramount importance for those whose dynamics are *always* in play.

Some folks within the BDSM community engage in their dynamic solely during a scene—whether publicly (e.g., in a dungeon space; at a kink party) or privately (e.g., within one's home; on vacation). Others, depending on setting and context, engage in their D/s dynamic more consistently throughout their day-to-day lives. No hard-set rules assert that D/s dynamics must exist at all times in all spaces. Fundamentally, whoever is engaging in the dynamic has the ability to negotiate the relationship structure as they see fit, which includes both the frequency and the intensity of the dynamic. While many kinky folks participate in situational BDSM, which occurs in specific situations or under specific circumstances, there are some individuals—albeit a much smaller number—whose D/s dynamic permeates their entire life. That's right: all day, every day.

"Total power exchange" (TPE) can be defined as a "socially constructed, consensual, full-time adherence to kink-related roles and behaviors untethered to time-limited scenes, woven into other life domains, and operating as an umbrella term to encompass 24/7 SM slavery, TPE, 24/7 D/s and other perpetual power dynamics" (Cascalheira et al., 2021). Heavily negotiated, this type of dynamic does not waver, whether or not the individual taking on the submissive role (s-type) is in the presence of their dominant partner (D-type) ("D-type" and "s-type" are utilized as umbrella terms to include the various dominant and submissive identities). Fundamentally, the weight of the hierarchy is always present and pre-negotiated rules dictate how the dynamic is integrated into all areas of life, which can include work life, home life, social life, and more. The day-to-day relationship within a 24/7 dynamic is grounded in rituals and behavioral patterns that continuously anchor the division of power between parties (Dancer et al., 2006). The thread of hierarchy remains tethered from one participant to the other(s); and for all participating individuals, that is precisely what they desire.

*⋆ **Content warning: The following section may be activating for those who have witnessed or experienced abusive relational dynamics. It may also be particularly difficult to read for those who have a history of disordered eating.***

I cannot stress enough that these dynamics should always be consensual, heavily negotiated, and frequently reassessed over time to ensure that they still serve the dynamic.★

There are several ways that the D-type can assert control over the s-type. These include but are not limited to the following:

- **Financial control:** When engaging in financial control, the D-type assumes total responsibility for overseeing and dictating the spending habits of the s-type, exerting influence over all financial decisions. The s-type willingly relinquishes control of their monetary resources to the D-type.
- **Decision control:** Decision control is characterized by the D-type assuming a central role in decision-making for the s-type. This involvement extends from everyday decisions, like the selection of clothing (see "Clothing control"), to pivotal life choices, such as determining where to live, whether to pursue formal education, or what jobs to apply for. Overall, by taking control of decisions, the D-type plays a crucial role in shaping the trajectory of the s-type's life.
- **Sexual control:** With the exception of pre-determined hard limits established during negotiations, the D-type assumes control over the dynamics of sexual interactions with the s-type. In some cases, blanket consent is granted to the D-type, affording them authority over the initiation, nature, and timing of sexual activities.
- **Sleep control:** When sleep control is established within a TPE dynamic, the D-type's authority extends to the regulation of not only bedtime but also morning and nighttime routines or rituals. Further, the D-type may utilize their influence to determine the duration of sleep for the s-type.
- **Bathroom/toilet control:** Within this dynamic, the D-type exercises control over if and when the s-type uses the bathroom. In some cases, particularly when forms of pet play or degradation are integrated into the dynamic, the D-type can also determine where the s-type may use the restroom (e.g., in the backyard or in a vessel other than a toilet). While this specific type of control requires the s-type to receive permission to use the restroom, negotiated exceptions may exist for times when the D-type may be unavailable (i.e., work, sleep, etc.).
- **Control over appearance:** Negotiating control over the s-type's appearance can take many forms, including but not

limited to choices regarding hair color and style, body modifications, physical activity, and the overall ways in which they present themselves. This type of control can be an umbrella that includes clothing, food, and sometimes exercise.

- **Clothing control:** A facet of control over appearance, within this dynamic, the D-type exercises full authority over decisions regarding the s-type's wardrobe. This encompasses selecting attire for various contexts, ranging from how they dress in the home to what is permitted as professional work attire, and outfits for community and social events. The way in which this type of control is integrated into the dynamic will change from relationship to relationship, sometimes being integrated as a set schedule (e.g., on Mondays, the s-type will wear X). In contrast, other times, the s-type will ask permission (whether in person or via text/photo/video call) once they have chosen an outfit they would like to wear.

- **Food control:** Food control is characterized not only by the D-type selecting what types of food the s-type consumes but also when and how that food is consumed. An example of asserting control over the way in which food is consumed is when pup play is integrated into the dynamic and the s-type is required to eat out of a dog bowl. While this type of control may be perceived as a form of punishment, in many circumstances, these are implemented to ensure the s-type is cared for and that their health remains a priority.

- **Exercise control:** Sometimes—although not always—considered an aspect of control over appearance, this type of control allows the D-type to dictate the nature, frequency, and intensity of the physical activities in which the s-type participates. Overall, this type of control can range from something as strict as a regimented exercise routine to simply ensuring that the s-type goes for a walk to get some fresh air each day.

- **Screentime control:** If the D-type chooses to initiate control over screen time, they will determine the extent of the s-type's engagement with electronic media, including television, phone, and computer access. The D-type may also choose to regulate the type of media the s-type consumes. An example of regulating media use is ensuring the s-type refrains from consuming media that contributes to issues of self-worth or insecurities. If the s-type has a job in which computer and phone access are required, the negotiated rules may not apply during work hours.

- **General time control**: An overarching form of control, the D-type may choose to determine how the s-type allocates and utilizes their time, influencing their daily schedules and activities. This can also include social control (see below).
- **Social control:** Social control involves the D-type asserting authority over the s-type's social interactions, influencing not only the individuals with whom the s-type engages but also the nature and timing of the social interactions.
- **Work/career control:** Work control includes the D-type assuming authority over the s-type's work and career choices. This includes decisions regarding not only the type of employment the s-type pursues but also if the s-type will work at all. This type of control may also include financial control (as listed above), where the D-type determines the manner in which earnings are utilized.

As you read the above list of potential types of control that can be implemented within a TPE relationship, you may have begun to wonder how this dynamic might play out in environments that may not be conducive to these types of expressions. Within 24/7 relationships, an essential aspect of negotiation includes determining the protocols for various life events. Thus, concerns around safety, privacy, and even legality are discussed, negotiated, and settled. Unlike the freedom to express one's dynamic that may exist in a dungeon space, there are many circumstances where it may not be safe to advertise the D/s dynamic (e.g., family gatherings, work events); thus, creative ways to maintain the thread of power exchange are often negotiated. A common example of creative negotiation is the requirement for an s-type to wear a necklace symbolic of their collar while in public settings and switch into their collar upon returning to a private setting. Other examples include setting up code words, symbols, and physical gestures, allowing secret communication in public spaces.

Lastly, and most importantly, it is critical to remember that any or all of these types of control are consented to by individuals pursuing this type of dynamic, and that this relationship structure should never arise due to duress, force, coercion, pressure, or guilt. Entering into this type of dynamic should be accompanied by a deep desire and commitment to the other, with each individual doing so with intention. These types of relationships may take months or even years to develop, and should be engaged in only after serious and deliberate consideration.

Due to the intense nature of 24/7 dynamics, it is essential that they are grounded in respect, empathy, self-awareness, flexibility, and honesty.

PERSONALITY TRAITS

"Sick," "perverted," "evil"—shall I go on? These are just a few of the many words that have been used to describe people who participate in BDSM. When a population has been both punished and harshly criticized—socially, medically, and legally—it is no surprise that when someone with no prior experience of participating in or learning about kink thinks about the characteristics of kinky people, they might conjure up an image or opinion based solely on stereotypical (yet inaccurate) depictions. One of the primary stereotypes about the kink community is that engagement in BDSM is a maladaptive coping mechanism resulting from past trauma or abuse. This viewpoint has been incredibly harmful to the kink community. It has undoubtedly impacted the ways in which healthcare professionals and the community at large engage with kinky people. Given this stereotype, it is unsurprising that much of the research around kink has looked at whether kink interests are indicative of some level of psychopathology—essentially looking for an answer to the question: are kinky people psychologically healthy? As more and more research began to be published, indicating time and time again that kinky people are psychologically well adjusted, the door began to open to more in-depth looks at the kink community. While the literature remains somewhat limited, the interest in understanding who kinky people are—rather than what they do or why they do it—has begun to garner much-needed attention.

In 2013, the first significant study seeking to understand the personality traits of BDSM practitioners was published, shedding important light on some of the central characteristics of kinksters—particularly those who identify as Doms, subs, and switches. This study was conducted by researchers Drs. Andreas Wismeijer and Marcel van Assen (2013), and looked at four components:

- the "Big Five" personality dimensions (openness to experience, conscientiousness, extroversion, agreeableness, neuroticism);
- attachment styles;
- subjective wellbeing; and
- rejection sensitivity.

The results of their study provided some of the first tools to begin chipping away at the negative perceptions of kinky people. For many years, the Wismeijer and van Assen study was the sole foundation for understanding kink personality features; and while a few studies have been conducted since then, due to the scarcity of personality-related research, there remains a lot to be uncovered.

> Regarding the major personality dimensions, our findings suggest that BDSM participants as a group are, compared with non-BDSM participants, less neurotic, more extraverted, more open to new experiences, more conscientious, yet less agreeable. BDSM participants also were less rejection sensitive, whereas female BDSM participants had more confidence in their relationships, had a lower need for approval, and were less anxiously attached compared with non-BDSM participants. Finally, the subjective well-being of BDSM participants was higher than that of the control group. Together, these findings suggest that BDSM practitioners are characterized by greater psychological and interpersonal strength and autonomy, rather than by psychological maladaptive characteristics.
>
> Wismeijer & van Assen, 2013

More recent research examined some of the same factors initially explored in the 2013 study and found conflicting results:

> These results are partly in line with, and partly contrary to, the results found by Wismeijer and van Assen (2013). The findings that are consistent with their study were the positive association between BDSM interest and openness to experience and the negative association between BDSM interest and agreeableness (only for women in our study). The findings that were not in line with Wismeijer and van Assen's (2013) study were the negative association between BDSM interest and conscientiousness and the finding that BDSM interest had no significant association with emotionality (neuroticism in the Big Five), extraversion, and agreeableness (for men).
>
> Paarnio et al., 2023

While researchers and academics continue to gain a better understanding of who kinky people are, there remains a significant gap in the research regarding the psychological characteristics of individuals who practice BDSM. However, due to the growing popularity of BDSM and the work of a variety of experts whose sole goals are understanding and seeking to enhance the lives of kinky folks, there is certainly hope that a deeper understanding of kinksters will soon be among us. Both of the studies discussed above ventured into new territory for kink research; and while further studies are necessary to gain an even better understanding of these particular traits within kink practitioners, the overall consensus is clear: kinky people either present with *more* favorable psychological characteristics than, or reflect *similar* psychological characteristics to, non-kinky people.

VARIATIONS ON D/S DYNAMICS

A sense of boundlessness and infinite possibility accompanies the kink experience, as identities are expansive and not necessarily fixed. One of the major complexities that can make kink expressions particularly tricky to grasp arises because of the many intersecting kink identities that one can hold. While some folks may refer to themselves strictly as a "Dominant" or a "submissive," others may tack on a variety of descriptors that indicate the type of dynamic they prefer, if their play involves pain or sensation, if a particular personality characteristic will show up, and more. Understanding the nuance of kink identity means remaining open to the ever-changing ways in which people embody their kink identities. Fundamentally, when discussing relational dynamics that are embedded in an agreed-upon hierarchy, one of the common points of confusion is understanding both the difference between a "Top" and a "Dominant," as well as a "bottom" and a "submissive." While these identities can indeed co-exist, the assumption is that they are always associated with one another is a prevalent misconception.

> The terms top, bottom, and switch generally refer to one's activity or role specifically during play or a scene. Hence, someone can refer to a person as a top ("She's a very good top") or refer to "topping" as a verb ("He topped me last weekend"). The same holds true for the terms bottom and switch. Those who identify as tops generally lead the interaction in a given scene, while those who identify as bottoms generally follow the interaction in a given scene.
>
> Simula, 2019

Understanding that "topping" and "bottoming" on their own refer to a leader/follower dynamic helps remove the potential assumption that all Tops are Doms and all bottoms are submissives. These leader/follower dynamics refer to the ways in which a particular kink interaction will go. While, from the outside, it may appear that one participant holds all of the power, this looks different from how an ownership/possession dynamic may look. As a quick refresher:

The terms dominant and submissive generally refer to roles or identities within consensual power exchange interactions or relationships. In such interactions or relationships, one partner—the dominant—takes control of the actions, behavior, appearance, and so forth of another partner—the submissive—within boundaries both individuals negotiate and agree on. People who switch within Dominant/submissive (D/s) relationships may switch within one relationship or may be dominant with one partner or partners and submissive with another/others. The terms Master and slave generally refer to roles or identities that are similar to those of Dominant and submissive but are often used in the context of relationships in which the consensual exchange of power encompasses more areas of life and/or the partners involved negotiate a greater depth of control for one partner than is common in D/s relationships. M/s relationships also tend to be understood as longer term commitments in comparison with D/s commitments, with some participants likening M/s to the BDSM version of a marriage.

Simula, 2019

This example—differentiating two potentially related but not guaranteed expressions—represents a much larger theme among the kink community: kink identities are individually based and can only fully be understood from the perspective of the individuals themselves. This is particularly important to remember as we begin

Scan the code to visit Kinkly's Dictionary of Sex Terms. Warning: Contains adult language and descriptions.

Figure 3.1   Kinkly Sex Terms (QR code)

uncovering the virtually unlimited variations of identity constellations. Being a Dominant, submissive, or switch indicates where within a power hierarchy a person may identify; and for some folks, this is the way in which they self-identify. The phrase "I am a submissive" is certainly valid. However, what happens when a submissive also loves pain—so much so that it is a part of the way they identify? In that case, the phrase "I am a masochistic submissive" may feel more aligned. (This is the part where taking a look at a glossary might come in handy.)

There are a variety of ways that BDSM identities can fuse together to encapsulate how someone self-identifies accurately. Identities may describe not only where within a hierarchy an individual likes to reside, but also a particular set of skills, such as a "rigger/rope Top" and a "rope bunny/rope bottom." Within this dynamic, bondage, in the form of rope tying, is integrated into the play (see Chapter 2 for a thorough explanation). There may not be any sexual engagement; and in many cases, the play may not fall within a power hierarchy. In those cases, this could be categorized as a leader/follower dynamic. The rigger is *leading* the scene, while the rope bunny *follows*. This is not to say, however, that this particular type of play cannot exist within an ownership/possession dynamic. Again, it is crucial to center the individual's self-identification rather than making any assumptions. To further explain—and hopefully not add to more confusion—D/s dynamics may also include some level of giving and receiving sensation (sadist/masochist); playfully pushing buttons or misbehaving (brat tamer/brat); utilizing financial domination to assert control (Findom/paypig) and many, many more. In addition to different types of D/s pairings, there are a variety of ways that folks can engage in D/s beyond TPE or scene-specific D/s. Educator Sarah Newbold describes a few more types of these dynamics below:

Long-distance D/s: In this arrangement, the Dominant and submissive maintain their power exchange dynamic despite being physically separated. They may use technology such as video calls, texting, or email to facilitate their DS interactions.

Switch D/s: In switch relationships, both people take on both dominant and submissive roles at different times or during different activities. The power exchange Dynamic can shift according to their desires and preferences.

Professional D/s: This type of relationship involves a financial transaction, with one person (usually a professional Dominant or submissive) providing D/s services to the other in exchange for payment.

Casual D/s: In casual D/s relationships, people may engage in power exchange dynamics without committing to a long-term or exclusive arrangement. They may have multiple D/s relationships or engage in D/s activities only occasionally.

Online D/s: Some people engage in D/s relationships exclusively online, using chat rooms, forums, or social media platforms to facilitate their power exchange dynamic.

Polyamorous D/s: In these relationships, one or more partners may be involved in multiple D/s connections with different individuals. The structure of these relationships can vary greatly, from hierarchical arrangements with a primary partner to more egalitarian, non-hierarchical configurations.

Role-specific D/s: In this form of D/s relationship, the power exchanged is limited to specific roles or scenarios, such as pet play, age play, or caregiver/little dynamics.

Newbold, 2023

The descriptions above allow us to understand further the importance of self-identification of kinky individuals and how they engage in their kink with one another. While we are covering many of the ways in which kink identities exist in a place of fluidity, we would be remiss to leave out the many ways in which non-monogamy and kink intersect. Due to limited research examining this particular intersection, "little is known about the prevalence and characteristics of people who engage in both kink and CNM" (Vilkin & Sprott, 2021). That said, within the few studies that have examined this dynamic, there appears to be a notable number of both kinky and non-monogamous folks within the samples. The following numbers represent three different studies and how/if their participants identified with or engaged in non-monogamy:

- **Study 1**: In this study of 1,580 kink-identified women, 39.9% were in poly or open relationships and 14.8% were monogamous (Rehor, 2015).
- **Study 2**: In this study of 50 participants, 80% were in non-monogamous relationships (Bauer, 2010).
- **Study 3**: In this study of 22 queer and poly-identified women, 65% were kink-poly identified (Deri 2015).

Fundamentally, kinky folks often hold more than one identity—certainly outside of the realm of kink, but often within their kinky lives as well. When exploring one's own identity or working with kinky folks in a clinical setting, it is crucial to explore *all* aspects of one's identity, leaving room for fluidity and expansiveness.

RISKS AND BENEFITS OF AUTHORITY EXCHANGE

As already mentioned, there are inherent risks built into kink play. In the same way that we put a seatbelt on while in a car, it is essential not only to remain aware of the risks related to kink play, but also to do what we can to minimize or mitigate those risks. Although a seatbelt does not completely eliminate the possibility of injury, it is a step in the direction of protecting oneself should anything go wrong. When it comes to authority exchange relationships—particularly those where playing with pain and sensation is integrated into the dynamic—being risk informed is absolutely critical. While the hope is that injuries will never occur during a kink scene—or really at any time in life—there is no way (aside from complete isolation, which I do not recommend) to avoid altogether the possibility that an error, mistake, or accident will occur resulting in an injury.

When it comes to playing with sensation and pain, BDSM participants have reported a number of injuries, both intentional and unintentional. These have included (but are not limited to) bruises, broken blood vessels, open wounds, abrasions, scrapes, broken bones, blood-borne pathogen exposure, fainting, and, in extremely rare cases, death (Drouin et al., 2023; Waldura et al., 2016; Schori et al., 2022). A 2021 study examined the literature on non-natural BDSM-related deaths and found that there had been 17 reported cases:

Strangulation in the course of erotic asphyxiation was the most common cause of death (88.2%). In 13 cases, a toxicology report for the deceased was mentioned, of which in eight cases (61.5%) toxicology analysis was positive. In four of these cases, the BDSM partner also tested positive for the same substance. Drugs or alcohol was involved in 64.3% of fatal BDSM play. In nine cases, the level of experience in BDMS activity of the deceased and the partner was described, and in all of them, the deceased and the partner were not new to BDSM play. Fatal outcomes of BDSM plays are rarer than autoerotic fatalities and natural deaths related to sexual activities.

Schori et al., 2022

While this type of research may seem jarring, it emphasizes the importance of introducing safeguards and participating in ongoing education. Although engaging in sexual activity in general can come at a risk, there are a variety of ways that these risks can be significantly minimized.

And while risks may be an inherent part of BDSM, there are also numerous benefits that one can experience from participating in kink. It can be counterintuitive to think about enhanced intimacy within an authority exchange relationship, but that thought typically arises due to the stereotypical assumptions about kinky folks based on depictions of kink in the media and personal internal conflict around kink participation. However, research suggests that engaging in a power exchange relationship can result in a heightened sense of relational closeness. In fact, studies have indicated that engagement in BDSM enhances aspects of sexual and relational intimacy, particularly as a result of a reduction of physical and psychological stress experienced through achieving an altered state of consciousness (Langdridge, 2007; Pitagora, 2017; Sagarin et al., 2003; Sagarin et al., 2015).

In addition to positive relational impacts, several studies have suggested a variety of personal benefits associated with kink participation. According to a 2016 study of 115 kink-oriented San Fransisco area residents, "a number of participants felt that their kink orientation had a positive effect on their health because it improved their general sense of well-being and encouraged them to take good care of themselves" (Waldura et al., 2016). Researchers have also discovered that BDSM practitioners may experience "relief from emotional strain, comprised mostly of depression, stress, and anxiety; relief of overload, mainly confusion, overwhelm and anger, and relief of social exclusion, made up mostly of disconnection and hiding parts of one's personality" (Silva & Mercury, 2015). The idea that BDSM participation influences a relief of social exclusion is consistent with both self-reports and research suggesting that community engagement is one of the primary benefits of being a part of the kink community. "People practicing BDSM often describe the BDSM 'community' as important to them because it adds meaning and offers security and a sense of belonging. Continuity and mutual recognition are arguably crucial factors in providing this sense of security." (Carlstrom, 2018)

Overall, kink-related literature suggests that engaging in kink can result in emotional relief, enhanced relaxation, relief from psychological stress, and increased awareness and introspection (Easton & Hardy, 2001; Newmahr, 2010; Barker, 2007). While these benefits may seem to suggest that kink participation can be a form of therapy, this belief can be hazardous and potentially dangerous. Although some of these positive impacts certainly do indicate the presence of a healing element that accompanies kink engagement, it is critical to remember that **kink is not therapy**. Kink may be therapeutic; it may be helpful in addition to therapy; but kink in and of itself is not therapy and nor should it be engaged with as such.

ADDITIONAL RESOURCES

The Heart of Dominance: A Guide to Practicing Consensual Dominance by Anton Fulmen

The Mistress Manual: The Good Girl's Guide to Female Dominance by Lorelei Powers

Different Loving: The World of Sexual Dominance and Submission by William Brame, Gloria Brame, and Jon Jacobs

Leading and Supportive Love: The Truth About Dominant and Submissive Relationships by Chris M. Lyon

BDSM Mastery Relationships: Your Guide for Creating Mindful Relationships for Dominants and submissives by Robert Rubel and Jen Fairfield

Where I am Led: A Service Exploration Workbook by Christina Parker

SADOMASOCHISM
Stefani Goerlich

Utilitarian philosopher Jeremy Bentham wrote, "[N]ature has placed mankind under the governance of two sovereign masters, pleasure and pain" (Bentham, 1780)—a full century before modern behavioral scientists started experimenting with classical conditioning, positive and negative reinforcements, and the way that sensory stimuli influence (or even control) the way we understand ourselves, our desires, and our place in the world. Bentham was a contemporary of the Marquis de Sade. Both men wrote their most influential works between 1789 and 1799; and while they were undoubtedly not colleagues, both men were deeply interested in the ideas of power, control, dominance, and authority. de Sade—after whom the very concept of sadism is named—explored themes of subjugation, imprisonment, and captivity in his writings of sexual conquest. For his part, Bentham—while certainly not an internationally infamous criminal libertine like de Sade—in some ways shared the latter's fascination with these topics. He is perhaps best known for his development of the Panopticon: a modern prison design that leveraged the prisoner's own uncertainty (in this case, regarding whether or not they were being watched) as a tool of control. In effect, Bentham proposed a form of institutional predicament play. While he was not a Sade-ist, Bentham—like de Sade—certainly understood the power of pain.

DOI: 10.4324/9781003312833-4

THE IDEA OF PAIN

Those who study Bentham's philosophy observe that:

> there are two forms of hedonism expressed in this seminal passage (quoted above): (1) psychological hedonism, which states that all motives of action are grounded in the apprehension of pain or the desire for pleasure; and (2) ethical hedonism, which holds that pleasure is the only good and actions are right in so far as they tend to produce pleasure or avoid pain.
>
> Crimmins, 2024

What, then, are we to make of those among us who experience pain as pleasure? Who seek it out or who eagerly mete it out to others? How should a clinician relate to, understand, and conceptualize their pain-seeking or pain-giving clients? Should sadism and masochism be understood as personality disorders, sensory processing differences, erotic diversities, dangerous aberrations, or perhaps some mix of all? These clients can be among the most challenging—even triggering—for the provider who encounters them. Moreover, much of this discomfiture lies in our personal, cultural, and theoretical understandings of the idea of pain.

In the West, we often talk about "pain and suffering." The two go hand in hand—to such a degree that the legal system recognizes that to inflict pain upon someone is to cause them to suffer. Within the law, "[p]ain and suffering refers to the physical discomfort and emotional distress that are compensable as noneconomic damages. It refers to the pain, discomfort, anguish, inconvenience, and emotional trauma that accompanies an injury" (Cornell Law School, 2020). This connection of pain with suffering can become a risk for sadomasochistic kinksters who find themselves facing legal scrutiny. However, our cultural discomfort with the notion of pain goes beyond the personal injury case law. We have entire fields of medicine devoted exclusively to mitigating and preventing pain. We have developed thousands of medications designed to erase our pain—many of which have been found over time to result in more horrific outcomes than the initial injury. Pain avoidance is a sign of wealth and affluence: "50% of the world's poorest populations live in countries that receive only 1% of the opioid analgesics distributed worldwide. By contrast, the richest 10% of the world's population live in countries that receive nearly 90% of the opioid pain relief medications" (Bhadelia et al., 2019). Our cultural relationship to the idea of pain is one of avoidance, aversion, and disapproval. Unlike other cultures around the world, we have not quite formed a clear understanding of the idea of pain with purpose.

PURPOSEFUL PAIN

In her book *Hurts So Good*, author and self-described masochist Leigh Cowart describes what she calls "pain on purpose": "the deliberate act of choosing to feel bad to then feel better" (Cowart, 2021). "Purposeful pain" (which Cowart uses interchangeably with "masochism") involves the strategic seeking out and application of various intense sensations to achieve an outcome (physiological, psychological, emotional, and/or spiritual) that the participants experience as beneficial. Cowart writes:

> Masochism is sexy, human, reviled, worshipped, and, at times, delightfully bizarre. From ballerinas dancing on broken bones to circus performers electrifying nails in their noses, to competitive eaters horking down peppers with escalating Scoville units, masochism is part of us. It's the people who grew up to become stunt performers, whose bruising connects them to their bodies in a way that makes them feel powerful. It's people who suffer from chronic pain and choose to find autonomy of their bodies by indulging in physical violence on purpose. It's the show Jackass and it's religious flagellation. It lives inside workaholics, piercing enthusiasts, and garden-variety pain sluts.
>
> Ibid

We have all had experiences where we have chosen purposeful pain. From navigating the emotional turmoil of ending a bad relationship to holding still through the sixth hour of a tattoo session to bearing down for one last push in order to bring a child into the world, there are moments in life when each of us recognizes that short-term suffering is the path toward a longer-term joy.

Even when our overall life circumstances are perfectly pleasant and entirely without discomfort, the addition of pain can serve to enhance our experience of pleasure. Researchers have identified nine specific biopsychosocial benefits associated with experiencing pain:

Pain enhances subsequent pleasure: Pain provides a contrast for pleasure, increasing the relative pleasantness of subsequent experiences.
Pain heightens sensory sensitivity: Pain heightens arousal and constrains attention on sensory experience, thereby increasing sensory receptivity.
Pain facilitates pleasure-seeking: Pain provides a justification for indulgence in pleasures that might otherwise arouse a sense of guilt.

Pain increases cognitive-affective control: Pain captures attention and brings cognitive resources online for effective problem-solving in response to the threat of pain.

Pain enables identity management: Pain promotes a physical experience of the self, thereby reducing high-level self-awareness and enabling identity change.

Pain demonstrates virtue: Pain may be interpreted as a symbolic test of a range of personal virtues.

Pain arouses empathy in others: The expression of pain increases empathy and arouses care and concern in others.

Pain increases relational focus: People seek social support in response to pain. Pain, therefore, provides a novel source of social connection with others.

Pain increases solidarity: Pain may be used to increase the value of relational ties with others, and shared pain may increase interpersonal bonding.

Bastian et al., 2014

Many of the benefits identified above have been observed both by other academics studying the psychology and physiology of pain on purpose and by members of the BDSM/kink community who write about their own lived experience of sadomasochism. The Science of BDSM Research Team at Northern Illinois University has published several studies exploring the ways our bodies physiologically respond not only to receiving pain but to giving it—offering scientific evidence for the relational focus and solidarity-building benefits

Scan the code for links to the Science of BDSM Team's published research.

Figure 4.1 The Science of BDSM Research (QR code)

identified by Bastian et al. Much of the work of Emma Sheppard, a disabled feminist kinkster and academic, focuses on the benefits of BDSM/kink for people who live with chronic pain—providing both research-based and experiential examples of the cognitive-affective control, identity management, and subsequent pleasure benefits in the list above. Sheppard specifically centers our understanding of the idea of eroticized pain and purposeful pain within the framework of intersectionality and crip studies:

> Pain, like all emotions, is shaped socially; our understandings of pain are social, as are our expressions; our understandings of pain are rooted in our gendered, racialized, sexualized identities—and others' readings of our bodyminds through those same prisms—and thus there is a need for understandings of chronic pain to be developed from crip sitpoints, to further develop a cripestemology of chronic pain.
>
> Sheppard, 2020

The role of pain as a driver of pro-social bonding and relationship building cannot be overstated for kinky people. In the same way that cultures around the world bring elements of pain into their religious and social rituals—from the Lakota (Sioux) Sun Dance to the Kavadi ritual of Hinduism; from traditionalist Catholics wearing a cilice under their business suit to the ritual whipping endured by Fulani adolescents entering adulthood in Benin—giving and receiving pain with purpose is a universal practice. As Sheppard rightly points out,

Scan the code to see a video of the Swami Temple Kavadi in 2022. Warning: Contains images of suspension piercing.

Figure 4.2   Swami Temple Kavadi (QR code)

we must understand our clients' relationship to pain (where one exists) as being yet another aspect of their intersectional identity; an aspect that can—and most likely will—change over time as their relationships evolve, their bodies experience ill health or decline, they experiment with body modification, or they explore BDSM/kink.

Even among BDSM practitioners who do not identify as sadists or masochists, a certain degree of chosen discomfort is often present within their relationship dynamics and their play. Whether this takes the form of tightly bound ropes or a degrading moniker, writing lines until the wrist cramps, or waiting in patient silence for what seems like (or is!) hours—discomfort for the sake of one's partner, one's pleasure, or one's service is a fairly standard element. These experiences serve not only to build the relational bond but to enhance the community bond as well. Showing off one's bruises with pride at the first munch after a scene can be a way to build rapport and bond with fellow community members. Moreover, this is true outside of the kink world as well. Researchers have found that people are more charitable after experiencing purposeful or communal pain—whether they received the painful stimuli themselves or not (Xygalatas, 2013). This research is particularly important when we consider the high degree of stigma experienced by sadomasochistic clients, the way that their desires (both to give and receive sensation) are pathologized, and the legal risks that they encounter when they act on these desires—even consensually. Unlearning the ways in which our cultural aversion to pain leads us down a path of kink-shaming and biased diagnostics is critical to our ability to do ethical work with sadomasochistic clients.

THE SADISM SPECTRUM

In order to work effectively with sadistic and sadomasochistic clients, we must be able not only to work within the framework of "pain with purpose," but also to understand that there are many purposes that pain might serve for our clients—including entirely nonsexual expressions of sadism. This is due in part to the fact that "sadism" is best understood not as a single, unified condition/desire/urge, but as a multidimensional descriptor ranging from healthy, adaptive, and pro-social to maladaptive, potentially dangerous, and antisocial. It is all too easy for the untrained to lean into pop culture tropes of sadists as evil and masochists as the butt of a joke. From *Criminal Minds* and *CSI* to *Family Guy* and 1970s-era "sexploitation" films, the most common portrayals of sadomasochism lean into extremes. This makes a certain degree of intuitive sense, since sadism has been linked to narcissism in many studies. It is important for the kink-affirming clinician to be mindful of the limitations of these studies and to recognize that most research on sadism is conducted using forensic and criminal populations, since these are among the few likely to be formally diagnosed with sexual sadism disorder—currently, the only form of sadism mentioned in the *Diagnostic and Statistical Manual of Mental Disorders*, Fifth Edition (*DSM-5*).

Sadistic personality disorder was a recognized diagnosis from 1987, when it was first included in the *DSM-III-R*, until 1994, when it was dropped from the *DSM-IV*. A proposal to include Milton's nonsexual sadism subtypes (explosive, spineless, enforcing, and tyrannical) in the *DSM-5* was considered but rejected (Paulhus & Dutton, 2016). Sexual sadism disorder, however, remains a diagnosis in both the *DSM-5* (where it is classified as a paraphilia) and the International Classification of Diseases, Tenth Edition (ICD-10); as does sexual masochism disorder, even though it is not uncommon for our sensation-seeking clients to enjoy both giving *and* receiving intense sensation (Greitemeyer, 2022). This narrow understanding of sadomasochism as two distinct and binary personality types, both of which are sexual in nature, exposes BDSM/kink practitioners to the risk of pathologizing and stigma—with potentially devastating consequences for those who receive formal diagnoses as sadists or masochists.

The criteria for diagnosing a client as either a sexual sadist or masochist are quite narrow. Our clients must experience intense, recurrent sexual arousal from either the physical or psychological suffering of others (sadism) or their own (masochism) for at least six months. These feelings must cause clinically significant distress for the client or impairment in functioning; and (for sadists) must have been acted on with a nonconsenting person (APA, 2013). These diagnoses are problematic since many otherwise well clients seek out the support of a therapist to help them process feelings of guilt and shame related to their sexual fantasies and desires. Ostensibly, a client who has struggled with sexual guilt or shame for longer than six months and whose internal conflict has begun to cause stress within their romantic relationships could theoretically be diagnosed with paraphilia. While we can hope that most clinicians would not make this leap, it has been the authors' experience that, far too often, a well-meaning but kink-uninformed clinician will note that "It's in the book!" (i.e., the *DSM*) and apply these highly stigmatizing diagnostic codes without due consideration or thoughtfulness.

> The DSM does not clearly distinguish between sexual deviance, sexual offending, and paraphilias. Sexual deviance is a moral construct that refers to sexual behaviors that contravene the mores of the particular society or culture. It is often equated with sexual abnormality, although this may reflect the general perception of what should be normal rather than what people really do.
>
> Yakeley & Wood, 2014

As a result, clinicians who lack an understanding of normative sexual expression and the prevalence of BDSM/kink specifically may apply an inaccurate and stigmatizing diagnostic code instead of a perhaps equally useful but less stigmatizing alternative. To accurately assess our non-forensic clients, we must have a clearer understanding of the sadism spectrum and use this to gauge our understanding of the unique set of circumstances each of our clients may be experiencing.

Pro-Social Sadism

This is a newer term developed to describe a phenomenon that researchers have observed within the BDSM community. Many self-identified sadists report that they are only able to experience arousal to sadistic stimuli when they are confident that the sadistic encounter is consensual. The notion of pro-social sadism is a crucial piece of the diagnostic puzzle for kink-affirming clinicians working in traditional settings, as well as those who may be engaged in forensic assessment and treatment. Because many of the common tools used to assess sexual sadism look only at checklists of behavior and do not assess for the level of consent desired, they can result in false positives for clients who are pro-social sadists—particularly when the client's erotica consumption or specific sensory desires (e.g., whipping, caning, edge play, breath play) is assessed in isolation from its greater context within BDSM/kink. Even when their desires may fall on the margins of what we deem socially acceptable—closer to de Sade's *120 Days* than James' *Fifty Shades*—the kink-affirming clinician should begin from the assumption that these fantasies are benign and engage in self-reflection regarding any potential countertransference that they may be experiencing in response to the sadistic desires being expressed.

> When assessing a client who fantasizes about or engages in high-risk/high-sensation forms of BDSM/kink, the clinician should focus on the role consent plays in these desires. Asking detailed questions, using Motivational Interviewing skills, and approaching erotic themes from a place of non-judgmental curiosity can allow the practitioner to gain insight into whether the client is engaging in negotiated consensual kink, visualizing a potential sexual/relational reality or rehearsing pathological behavior.
>
> Goerlich, 2024

Marking this distinction within our case conceptualizations for sadistic kinksters is crucial because it allows us to hold space for consent even within role-played behavior that can appear non-consensual on the surface.

> The meanings applied to acts, behaviors, and fantasies as powerful or submissive draw on their meanings from histories and experiences from social life . . . fantasy allows us to suspend the familiar in a way that can allow us to sink deeper into it, thus gaining insights which are nearly impossible to attain when we go about our lives "as usual."
>
> Toth, 2015

As we move along the sadism spectrum, we will encounter darker, more problematic sadistic possibilities that are not predicated on consent. We will see how, as Toth puts it, the sadistic personality can move from play to practice.

Empathetic Sadism

Fritz Breithaupt describes "empathetic sadism" as "the emotional and intellectual enjoyment that most people feel in situations of altruistic punishment, watching tragedies, and such common events as embarrassment, bullying, and domination" (Breithaupt, 2019). The cathartic experience of watching a horror movie when one is in a bad mood and feeling one's mood lighten as each hapless victim falls is one example of empathetic sadism. Empathetic sadism has not received nearly the same amount of research attention as everyday sadism (see below) and its more pathological siblings, but it deserves mention as one iteration of sadism that may be far more common than the data might indicate. Because nearly all research on sadism is conducted on forensic populations, we do not have much information about how common the sub-pathological variants, such as empathetic sadism, might be—in our clients *and* ourselves.

Even as we work to assess and contextualize our clients' feelings and desires into a cohesive case concept, we must also be mindful of the reactions that might be evoked for us in these encounters. Particularly when our client engages in behavior or expresses desires/ fantasies that we have personal ethical or moral struggles with, we must be aware of our capacity for wielding the very tools of therapy as an instrument of empathetic sadism.

> In her attempt to reach the patient, to reinstate herself as an active agent and subject, and also to dislodge the patient from a rut of despair, passivity, or malignity, the analyst may escalate to a sadistic response, even if she suspects that this might cause the patient pain.
>
> Csillag, 2014

One way this sadistic response could manifest is through our diagnostic process when a clinician feels justified or even righteous in applying a "harsh" label, such as a paraphilic disorder, to a client in an effort to punish them for falling outside of what is normal for their time and place. Research has shown that reaching biased conclusions by ignoring conflicting information causes our brain's reward center to activate (Westen et al., 2006). In other words, we experience pleasure when we convince ourselves we are right. This may explain the connection between altruistic (e.g., "deserved") punishment and the enjoyment experienced by empathetic sadists. There are many ways this could present in the therapeutic relationship: a sense of pleasure when the client experiences consequences for their problematic behavior; pride; or self-satisfaction when a therapeutic observation results in an emotional response such as tears.

Another form this can take is through what Breithaupt calls "empathetic vampirism":

> The empathizer feels and experiences the world vicariously via others and thereby participates in their fate without having their best interests in mind. Instead, the implicit interest of the empathizer lies in his or her own act of experiencing. The other becomes a medium of one's experience. Even in cases where the empathizer imagines having the best interests of the other in mind—the results may prove otherwise.
>
> Breithaupt, 2018

In the same way that we must be aware of our capacity for empathetic sadism, the kink-affirming clinician must take care that they are not engaging in acts of empathetic vampirism—engaging with their client's kink identities or disclosures about BDSM as a way to feed their own voyeuristic emotional needs. Failing to recognize our capacity for emotional vampirism—particularly when working with trauma survivors, as well as gender, sexuality, and relationship minorities—exposes both ourselves and our clients to the potential for harm.

Everyday Sadism

For many, the 18th-century aristocrat Marquis de Sade is inseparable from the disorder which bears his name. Known for his violent erotic writings, de Sade spent most of his adult life in various European prisons and asylums because of the content and themes of his novels and diaries. His writings are horrific to many and have been banned off and on throughout Europe and the Americas over the last three centuries (Phillips, 2005). What is most salient to our point here is that, as gruesome as his tales are for many readers—both now and during his lifetime—they were not terribly far off from similar practices that were commonplace at the time he was writing:

> These works described a vast range of violent and sexual acts, including rape and murder. However, they were produced at a violent time, when public executions of quartering and other torturous methods were used and were popular. Block, a psychiatrist who studied Sade's life and works, concluded that "the works of Marquis de Sade drip with the blood of his century."
>
> Toth, 2015

In other words, the Marquis de Sade might have been an everyday sadist.

> Everyday sadism is defined as a pleasure-driven form of aggression demarcated by having an enjoyment of cruelty in normal, everyday situations. Everyday sadists have lower levels of disgust sensitivity, demonstrate willingness to harm bugs, experience reward when doing so, and demonstrate a willingness to implement unprovoked aggression towards an unknown other. Everyday sadism positively predicts . . . enjoyment of internet trolling, behavioural delinquency in boys, rape myth acceptance and sexual violence in men, hostile femininity . . . and adversarial sexual attitudes in women.
>
> Erickson & Sagarin, 2021

Everyday sadists are those who may have a strong desire to cause misery to others but who lack the impulse to act out these desires in ways that are likely to disrupt their own lives and relationships. "Instead of seeking to alleviate suffering, these individuals may seek opportunities to exercise brutality and indulge their appetites for cruelty" (Buckels et al., 2013). Everyday sadists act on their desires through violent video games or aggressive contact sports; by taking on employment that lets them exercise power over others in ways that leave them feeling (non-sexually) dominant over those they encounter; or by engaging in acts of petty cruelty and meanness that distress those who experience them but fall below pathological or criminal levels of harm. Unlike pathological sadists, everyday sadists can self-regulate and control their behavior when they choose to do so and are unlikely to experience distress about their actions. Like de Sade's writings, everyday sadism is informed by its time and place, and is both culturally and socially contextual. One example of this socio-cultural context can be found in the act of dog fighting. When NFL quarterback Michael Vick was convicted of animal cruelty after being caught running an illegal dogfighting ring that resulted in injury and death to dozens of dogs, one of the defenses offered by Vicks' supporters at the time was that this was a "sport" rooted in Vick's rural Southern upbringing (ALDF, 2010)—a cultural difference rather than an act of cruelty.

Everyday sadists may present as mid-level bureaucrats or barroom brawlers. They can be high-profile litigators or stay-at-home parents. They may be verbally cutting and cruel or engage in petty actions that cause low-level harm and discomfort to those needing assistance. They enjoy holding power and wielding it over others. They are more likely to score higher in psychopathy, Machiavellianism, and narcissism than their non-sadistic peers (Buckels, 2018). Everyday sadism may also be comorbid with pathological altruism, which we will discuss in greater detail in the next section of this chapter.

Sexual Sadism Disorder

Sexual sadism disorder—the only piece of the spectrum that is currently listed in the *DSM-5*—has a very specific, very limited application. It is ideally intended to diagnose sexual sadism that *causes harm*, either because the client has enacted their fantasies on a non-consenting partner or because they are themselves experiencing significant distress due to their desires. This standard is somewhat nebulous and leaves a great deal open to interpretation by the clinician—an interpretation that is confused somewhat by the *DSM-5*'s conflation of sexual sadism with BDSM (APA, 2013). This confusion is exacerbated by some of the screening tools that have been developed to assess sexual sadism disorder within forensic contexts. The Severe Sexual Sadism Scale (SSSS), for example, is considered a "reliable and valid" assessment of sexual sadism disorder—and yet because it was developed using a sample of 105 sex offenders (Mokros et al., 2012), it includes many criteria that may result in a false positive for consensual BDSM practitioners. The SSSS is scored by calculating the total number of "yes" responses from the list below. A score of 7 is seen to be a good indicator of the presence of sexual sadism disorder.

> Offender is sexually aroused by sadistic acts.
> Offender exercises power/control/domination over victim.
> Offender humiliates or degrades the victim.
> Offender tortures victim or engages in acts of cruelty on victim.
> Offender mutilates sexual parts of victim's body.
> Offender engages in gratuitous violence of wounding towards victim.
> Offender keeps records (other than trophies) or trophies (e.g. hair, underwear, ID).
> Offender mutilates nonsexual parts of victim's body.
> Victim is abducted or confined.
> Evidence of ritualism in offense.
> Insertion of object into bodily orifices.
>
> Nitschke, Osterheider, & Mokros, 2009

Because the SSSS scale and other similar tools were not developed with input from the mainstream BDSM community, they include criteria that many kinksters would agree apply to them—such as exercising power/control/domination or engaging in humiliation/degradation. Interestingly, the SSSS does not consider consent a variable at all—it is a binary yes/no checklist of behaviors used by outside observers to "rate" the factors they can observe. It does not ask whether these activities were negotiated at all or enjoyed by the receiver (here called the "victim"). Some of the language ("gratuitous," "cruelty") is subjective, which exposes consensual kinksters to risk of legal scrutiny if and when they need to seek medical assistance after a scene and puts them at risk of prosecution or incarceration for otherwise consensual (if perhaps edgier or higher-risk) BDSM play. Indeed, much of the language used when conceptualizing a standard for sexual sadism is forensic in nature—describing (as we see above) the participants as "victims" and "offenders" or drawing parallels between sexual sadism and "lust murderers" (Longpre et al., 2016).

Is not to say that sadistic crime does not exist or that sexual sadism cannot be pathological in nature. However, we must recognize the limited usefulness of our current forensic understanding of sexual sadism when generalized to the broader population that most clinicians work with. When we understand sexual sadism as *only* being maladaptive, abusive, and harmful, we run the risk of pathologizing clients whose desires should not be understood as problematic. "SM (sadomasochism) can serve as an outlet for those who seek pain/pleasure experiences. In particular, SM can provide a safe space for players to experience and exert control upon another . . . such behaviors can be transformative and spiritually fulfilling" (Worthen, 2022). Kink-affirming clinicians acknowledge that pathological behaviors exist. What they do not do is rush to assume that behaviors are pathological simply because they are non-normative. There remains a serious gap in our assessment toolbox for kinky clients; and as long as we continue to develop assessment instruments that draw only from the experiences of forensic populations, we will continue to create both clinical and institutional systems that are biased against erotic minorities.

Sadistic Personality Disorder

Sadistic personality disorder (SPD) is a controversial diagnosis that is not officially recognized within the *DSM*. It was included in the *DSM-III-R* in a section titled "Proposed Diagnostic Categories Requiring Further Study" but was ultimately removed from the *DSM-IV-TR*. SPD is differentiated from antisocial personality disorder (discussed briefly in the next section) by its relationship to power and control:

> Unlike antisocial or other disorders relating to violence or illegal behavior, sadistic personality disorder was distinguishable in that their actions were meant primarily to gain pleasure or achieve dominance and control, rather than primarily for profit or due to the need to cope with stressors. Sadists also were differentiated in that their violence occurred not under extreme emotional states or in the context of seeking financial gain, but rather for the pursuit of pleasure, control, or satisfaction.
>
> Levesque, 2018

SPD is often conflated and may present concurrently with another commonly used yet unrecognized diagnostic term—"psychopathy":

> Psychopathy, while not a formal diagnosis, is a personality disorder in which the individual displays a lack of conscience, seeks self-gratification

at others' expense, is emotionally detached, and generally leaves a path of destruction in the wake of their interpersonal relationships.

Murphy & Vess, 2003

It is clear that the mental health field struggles to accurately and fairly describe people and personalities that are cruel, violent, self-serving, and destructive. One of the challenges to creating an accurate taxonomy of beyond-the-pale behaviors is the subjective and ever-shifting society in which these behaviors occur. As Block pointed out, even de Sade's writings were indicative (to a point) of his own time and place. Our understanding of power and control, pain versus cruelty, and mental illness versus moral choice is rooted in cultural norms and personal values that can play out on subconscious levels within the minds of the clinician, the client, and (in worst-case scenarios) the courts. Much of the spectrum we have explored over the last few pages is rooted in the psychological theory of personality development. We have not begun to touch on (nor do we have the space to explore) the roles that hormones and neurotransmitters, environmental factors, early childhood attachment, operant conditioning, and cognitive schemes play in the choices our clients make about how they move through the world, interact with their partners and others, and explore and experience pain and other sensations (Vandiver & Braithwaite, 2022). Engagement with intense sensations can look and feel concerning to the outside observer. That is why we must be so judicious in how we approach our sadomasochistic clients—both in the assessment tools we use when diagnosing them and in the words we choose when interacting with them. Let us explore the latter further.

PAIN VERSUS SENSATION

As we have discussed, one of the reasons why some clinicians struggle with sadomasochistic clients is the fact that the idea of pain is a negative one in many Western cultures. Our cultural understanding of the necessity of pain and the role it should play in life influence and inform the way we respond (both externally and internally) to clients who include pain play in their erotic and relational lives (Peacock & Patel, 2008). For some, pain is an experience to be stoically endured as a demonstration of one's strength and capacity for resilience. Others may interpret pain through the lens of their spiritual or religious traditions—seeing pain as a punishment, a sacrifice, or a form of karma. In America and Europe, for the most part, pain is medicalized: something to be avoided (Jensen et al., 2017), mitigated (Brennan et al., 2007), or cured entirely (Price & Gold, 2018). There are few opportunities to experience "positive pain" in our highly medicalized culture—childbirth, tattoos, and intense exercise being the most common. The idea that someone might embrace pain as a positive force in their lives and relationships can bring up many of the same biases or negative stereotypes that we have discussed throughout this chapter, especially since we are hardwired to associate pain as a physiological warning signal. "Of the various consequences our actions can have, pain is probably the strongest indicator that our behavior needs adjustment . . . Pain therefore motivates decisions and actions to prevent future harm" (Wiech & Tracey, 2013).

The kink-affirming clinician may choose to shift their language to avoid these potential biases. By using the term "sensation" rather than "pain," we can acknowledge the experiences that our clients enjoy about sadomasochistic play without using the potentially stigmatizing/biased language of pain. "Sensation" is a value-neutral way to describe the same physiological reactions that sadomasochistic play can evoke for the kinky client. It also opens up the clinical dialog to allow space for the client to label and define their own experiences without outside voices applying their own descriptors. "Sensation" also creates opportunities for the clinician to guide the kinky client through somatic exploration of their emotional experiences as well. We can acknowledge that strong feelings are experienced physically and emotionally and encourage the client to observe and tie threads between their positive and negative emotional states and potential corollary physical experiences. Psychoeducation about the physiology of emotions can be a powerful form of normalization for kinky clients, giving them greater insights into their own emotional reactions and sensory desires. By using terminology such as "sensation" rather than "pain," we reframe our client's experiences to honor the truth of their desires while feeling less judgmental or problematic to them and ourselves. For clients who may seek therapeutic support due to fear that their sadomasochistic desires are unhealthy or pathological, using the language of sensation can open doors to conversation and clinical education about pro-social sadism and the personal and relational benefits for those who engage with it.

DIFFERENTIAL DIAGNOSTICS

When considering the practices, behaviors, and relationship dynamics that fall under the umbrella of sadomasochistic play, it is important that the clinician balance being affirming and supportive our clients' erotic identities, agency, and personal risk framework with our own ethical need to be cleareyed about the potential risks of intense sensation play. We have discussed the fact that "there is no evidence that BDSM practitioners in general suffer from any particular form of psychological disturbance and in fact . . . seem to be mentally and emotionally well-adjusted" (Richters et al., 2008). That fact is clear. We have also discussed the ways in which seemingly problematic behaviors can be expressed in emotionally healthy ways. The vast majority of BDSM/kink practitioners engage in safety-aware, consensual, negotiated play. For just a few pages, however, let us explore the possibilities that exist when problematic—or even dangerous—behavior is mistaken for consensual kink.

Pathological Altruism

Psychoanalyst Emmanuel Ghent proposed a distinction between what we clinically call "masochism" and what he termed "surrender." His concept of surrender as "a quality of liberation and expansion of the self as a corollary to the letting down of defensive barriers" (Ghent, 1990) is one that resonates with many kink people and ties nicely in with Roy Baumeister's concept of masochism as "escape from self." At their core, the terms "sadism," "masochism," and "sadomasochism" are clinical labels that the BDSM community has adopted. As such, they carry specific pathologizing connotations that other community-generated terms—such as "owner"/"property," "caregiver"/"little," or "hedonist"—do not. Ghent goes on to observe that "it is this passionate longing to surrender that comes into play in at least some instances of masochism" (ibid).

One of the risks within sadomasochistic play is the potential for this desire to become maladaptive: to move beyond the flow state of ecstatic surrender described by Baumeister (and measured by Sagarin et al., 2009), and morph into something more akin to pathological altruism. "Pathological altruism", as proposed by author and researcher Barbara Oakley, is "an evolutionary oxymoron . . . Altruism is underpinned by traits and behaviors, such as empathy, that evolved to help us humans function smoothly together. But . . . sometimes our well-meaning attempts to help others can make matters worse . . . (it is) selflessness gone awry" (Habash, 2011). Brent Turvey identifies "masochistic altruism" as one specific variant that is relevant to our discussion of differential diagnoses:

> Masochistic altruism . . . refers specifically to a maladaptive need to suffer or be the victim, compensating for profound envy, jealousy, anger, aggression, and/or low self-esteem and thoughts of inadequacy. Masochistic altruists seem to be characterized by a pattern of self-sacrifice in which altruism is a coping mechanism for masking inner negativity and conflict . . . Masochistic altruism often involves the conscious or subconscious belief that one does not deserve to be happy.
>
> Turvey, 2012

This self-loathing is distinct from the guilt and shame that some kinky people experience about their desires; however, it can result in some people engaging in BDSM activities that would otherwise fall outside of their personal boundaries/limits as a way of processing their feelings or working through this internal conflict. While there is some evidence that BDSM play can have therapeutic benefits as a form of reclamation and reprocessing for kink-identified clients (Goerlich, 2023), the clinician must exercise good judgment, affirmational curiosity, and motivational interviewing to help clients identify and evaluate their particular masochistic motivators.

"Like all forms of sexual behavior, kinky sex can be enlisted in the service of neurotic or self-destructive forces, and it is not always easy to distinguish between positive and negative expressions of sex" (Nichols, 2011). The kink-affirming clinician can assess for masochistic altruism by being mindful of instances when the client:

- expresses an unwillingness or aversion to the activities they are engaging in;
- makes statements that indicate they do not believe they are worthy of setting limits or having boundaries;
- states that their desire to please their partner is greater than their desire for BDSM/kink play;
- expresses concern that if they do not engage in certain activities/ dynamics, their partner will leave them or spend more time with another;
- states that they "deserve" mistreatment or punishment for who or what they are;

- does not experience pleasure or joy in power exchange, or views it as an obligation, punishment, or commentary on their identity and value; and/or
- is fearful that saying no to a specific act or role will brand them as undesirably "vanilla."

It is entirely possible to be strong, self-possessed, and self-affirming, and also desire submission or surrender. Author and memoirist Anaïs Nin wrote of herself:

> I do not want to be the leader. I refuse to be the leader. I want to live darkly and richly in my femaleness. I want a man lying over me, always over me. His will, his pleasure, his desire, his life, his work, his sexuality the touch-stone, the command, my pivot. I don't mind working, holding my ground intellectually, artistically; but as a woman, oh, God, as a woman I want to be dominated. I don't mind being told to stand on my own two feet, not to cling, be all that I am capable of doing, but I am going to be pursued, fucked, possessed by the will of a male at his time, his bidding.
>
> Nin, 1992

Healthy power play—whether it takes the form of a power-exchange relationship or a one-time sensory exploration scene—facilitates a liberating sense of surrender for the person on the receiving end. Whether this surrender is termed "subspace" (Scott, 2015), "over-whelm" (Saketopoulou, 2023), or "flow" (Ambler et al., 2017), it should be experienced by the parties involved as consensual, pleas-urable (if not comfortable), and affirmational. Where we have cause for concern that our client is engaging in any behavior—sexual, rela-tional, substance, or otherwise—out of a desire to repudiate or pun-ish some aspect of themselves, the kink-affirming clinician will work to encourage the client to challenge distorted cognitions, develop a healthy ego, and build the skills necessary to set clear boundaries for their lives, their bodies, and their relationships.

Self-harm

It is a common clinical misconception that sadomasochistic play is a form of self-harm or self-injury. Much like masochistic altruism, the motivations for engaging in self-harming behaviors are quite differ-ent from the reasons why one might choose to engage in consensual sadomasochistic play. Persons who engage in acts of self-harm—which can take forms ranging from cutting or burning themselves to snapping a rubber band repeatedly against their skin and many acts in between—are typically doing so as a way to cope with or release strong emotions; to externalize their internal distress; to feel a sense of control over their lives or circumstances and for many other reasons (NHS, 2023). Persons who engage in self-harm are more likely to be experiencing social difficulties and/or mental health concerns than their non-self-harming peers (Townsend et al., 2015). Self-harming behaviors have also been linked to suicidal ideation and increased risk of suicidality.

In contrast, research has found that BDSM engagement is not significantly related to higher psychological distress (Richters et al., 2008); while those engaging in BDSM have attachment styles which are "almost identical" to those of the general population (Sandnabba et al., 2002), and have higher subjective wellbeing than their non-kinky peers (Wismeijer & van Assen, 2013). Although both BDSM and self-injury can result in intense physical sensation (including pain) and may leave injurious marks upon the receiver, the crucial difference between these two behaviors is the intent behind them. In the same way that kinky submission/surrender is not the same as masochistic altruism, sadomasochistic play (even solo play) under most circumstances is not the same as self-harm.

> When asked the difference between self-harm as a coping mechanism and BDSM practices, every participant replied with the word "intent"... Although BDSM practitioners use consensual pain as pleasure, the vast majority of participants agreed that self-harming falls in a completely separate category due to self-awareness . . . BDSM meets this need in a different, safe, and managed way.
>
> Afana, 2021

BDSM/kink practices can certainly be utilized as a way to sublimate maladaptive impulses or desires and channel these into risk–aware, consensual, mutually pleasurable activities. Early research has shown that kinky trauma survivors specifically experience a powerful sense of reclaiming and reprocessing through their BDSM practice. It is possible for clients with histories of self-harm to find a healthier outlet for those impulses within the world of consensual sadomasochistic play. The role of the kink-affirming clinician is to have open and ongoing conversations about the emotional drivers behind this play, the cognitive distortions that may (or may not) exist for the client, and the broader set of emotional coping skills each client has to choose from.

Antisocial Personalities

On the topic of harm and intent, we must acknowledge that within every community, bad actors exist. These bad actors exploit the in-group trust of marginalized communities in order to access potential victims.

> Victims of crime and abuse are disproportionately represented by marginalized communities, where the relationship with law enforcement is already tense. When a crime is committed against someone from these communities, they likely have an existing distrust and skepticism that they will be believed and protected by the system.
>
> Dunn, 2023

For the BDSM/kink community, historical experiences of discrimination from institutional systems such as law enforcement personnel, family courts, and mental health providers increase the risk of harm by those who adopt the language, symbols, and mannerisms of BDSM culture in order to build rapport and access otherwise private spaces where their victims can be found. Concerns about SPD being used as a psychological rationalization for offending behaviors was one factor that led to the removal of the diagnosis from the *DSM*. Likewise, coercive paraphilic disorder was considered and excluded due to concerns that it would be used to rationalize sexual assault as a behavioral problem rather than a criminal offense (Toth, 2015). These concerns are validated when one considers that there have been several high-profile cases where BDSM/kink has been used as a defense following violent crimes ranging from rape (AAP, 2018) to manslaughter (Price, 2023) to intimate partner violence-related homicide (O'Toole, 2015). One of the ways that the BDSM/kink community has coordinated to protect its members from unethical bad actors is through the implementation of local whisper networks and online black lists to warn one another away from negative encounters or problematic/dangerous individuals (Clark-Flory, 2012). These resources are both important for protecting kinky people from harm and controversial in their implementation—particularly when someone feels that they have been falsely accused or unfairly added.

We have explored the spectrum of sadistic behaviors and motivations at length already, but one group has not yet been addressed: antisocial personalities. Before SPD was removed from the *DSM-IV*, researchers sought to gain insights into what disorders were commonly co-occurring in individuals who had been diagnosed with SPD. 42.1%

of the study subjects who had been labeled as sadistic personalities were also diagnosed with antisocial personality disorder (Berger et al., 1999). Antisocial personality disorder—which is colloquially (and somewhat inaccurately) used interchangeably with "psychopathy" in much of the popular literature—is characterized by "deficits in emotional functioning . . . superficial charm, irresponsibility, fearlessness, conning behavior/manipulation, and lack of empathy" (Lobbestael et al., 2023). While psychopathy is not a formal diagnosis within the *DSM-5-TR* or ICD-10, it is a term commonly used within forensic psychology and the world of criminal justice. It has been linked to antisocial personality disorder in part due to the Hare Psychopathy checklist tool, which divides the observed traits into interpersonal and antisocial factors (Vandiver & Braithwaite, 2022).

In working to differentiate antisocial traits from pro-social sadism, it can be beneficial for the kink-affirming clinician to have working knowledge of the ongoing dialog around how best to identify, assess, and conceptualize clients with sadistic or psychopathic traits. As with any population, we must take care to recognize that simply having a specific set of behavioral criteria or personality traits does not mean that a client is dangerous to themselves or others. In recent years, a number of popular works have been written by individuals who meet the criteria for psychopathy who live healthy, adaptive, and harm-free lives—including one neuroscientist who discovered his own psychopathy when his own brain scans were inadvertently included in the data set of a study he was conducting on the brain scans of serial killers (Stromberg, 2013). The concept of fearless dominance may help us bridge the conceptual gap between pro-social sadists, everyday sadists, and psychopaths or antisocial personalities.

Fearless dominance is hallmarked by "interpersonal potency, physical fearlessness, risk-taking, and calmness in the face of danger" (Lilienfeld et al., 2016). You may already be noticing some commonalities between fearless Dominants and our kinky sadomasochists. While fearless dominance is often associated with psychopathic or antisocial personalities, "when one burrows down more deeply . . . [it] is largely unassociated with three of the four facets of the PCL-R (the Hare Psychopathy checklist)" (ibid). Additionally, fearless dominance is associated (weakly but positively) with attributes such as heroism and altruism. In other words, pro-social sadism and fearless dominance might have enough in common to be misrecognized as psychopathy by clinicians lacking sufficient clinical skill. Let us end this section by noting that neither sadists nor fearless Dominants should be assumed to be antisocial personalities based on behavioral traits alone. The *DSM* makes it clear that antisocial personality disorder is diagnosed only when there "is a pervasive pattern of disregard for, and violation of, the rights of others that begins in childhood or early adolescence and continues into adulthood" (APA, 2013). Even kink-affirming clinicians will encounter clients whose fetishes, sensory play, or relationship dynamics make them uncomfortable. Be wary of inadvertently diagnosing your own discomfort by applying clinical labels that may not accurately reflect the client's behavioral intent. Bad actions absolutely exist within the BDSM/kink community—as they do in all communities. But kinky people are no more likely to be bad actors by virtue of their kinks than a neuroscientist is to be a criminal simply because of their brain.

RISKS AND BENEFITS

Humanity's evolutionary aversion to pain can limit our appreciation for the potential benefits that some sensation-seeking clients experience. Intense sensation can facilitate learning, encourage adaptation, foster empathy and altruism, and contribute to personal growth, appreciation for life, and resilience (Bastian et al., 2014). Kinky clients specifically may report enhanced relationship closeness (Sagarin et al., 2009); stress reduction and/or cathartic relief (ibid); increased serotonin levels (Kekatos, 2017); increased sense of body awareness and sensory experience (Turley, 2016); improved self-esteem and body confidence (Martinez, 2016); increased sense of personal resilience (Damm et al., 2017); psychological release (Baumeister, 1988); an outlet for processing unhealthy desires (Hammers, 2014); and increased/improved communication between partners (Kleinplatz, 2006), among other potential benefits.

This is not to say that sadomasochistic play does not carry a degree of risk. As we have discussed throughout this book (and will explore in depth in Chapter 9), any physical activity carries with it some risk. Likewise, entering into any close, vulnerable relationship with another person (or persons) also opens us up to psycho-emotional risk. The chances we take when we open ourselves up to another are part of the romanticism of falling in love: we cannot experience the highs without exposing ourselves to the potential for hurt as well.

I define vulnerability as uncertainty, risk in emotional exposure. With that definition in mind, let us think about love. Waking up every day and loving someone who may or may not love us back, whose safety we cannot ensure, who may stay in our lives or may leave without a moment's notice, who may be loyal to the day they die or betray us tomorrow—that's vulnerability.

Brown, 2012

The kink-affirming clinician must pause to acknowledge the risk that is intrinsic in *all* interactions with others—both physical and emotional as well as sexual—when conceptualizing risk for sadomasochistic clients because we run the risk ourselves of centering concerns over physical safety and potential for harm ahead of all other risk factors. This represents a bias against sensory play and can sometimes result in clinicians prioritizing physical risk ahead of the other equally impactful factors that our clients may need to consider. When this occurs, we are in danger of being perceived as paternalistic or kink-shaming by our sadomasochistic clients rather than curious or risk-aware.

This is not to say that the clinician can ignore all risks in the name of being kink-affirming and non-shaming. Indeed, we must acknowledge that the clinician themselves must be aware of the risk of improper diagnoses or inadequate treatment planning when working with sadistic or sadomasochistic clients. While the vast majority of BDSM practitioners who engage in intense sensory play fall within the category of pro-social sadists—those for whom sensation play is enjoyable only when it is unambiguously consensual—it is possible in rare instances for the clinician to encounter someone whose desires fall outside of this cohort. Jemma Toth recounts a scenario that is relevant to our discussion of sadomasochistic risk:

I have analysed a case study that involved the rape and murder of a young woman. The woman identified as being a sexual masochist and was role-playing her rape and murder with a partner, who identified as a sexual sadist. However, their relationship went beyond role-play when he completed the act of murder. This relationship is one example of the difference between sexual fantasy and visualizing reality. The difference between this woman who fantasized about being murdered, but didn't want to die, and her partner who ultimately killed her, was that during their sexual relationship, she was playing, while he was practicing.

Toth, 2015

The risk for kink-affirming clinicians who are working with clients who enjoy extreme forms of play—such as consensual non-consent, breath play, knife/edge play, humiliation, or dehumanization—is that we may underestimate the degree of risk due to our own inclinations to avoid appearing kink-shaming or our tendency to emphasize the benefits of kink. It is imperative that clinicians who work primarily with BDSM practitioner clients—and are therefore more likely to encounter clients who fall within what Richard Sprott and Anna Randall call "playing with dark emotions" (TASHRA, 2023)—continue to engage in peer consultation, cultural competency continuing education, and ongoing training in clinical assessment and kink-affirming safety planning. If one does not work primarily with BDSM/kink-identified clients, understanding one's own level of competency and having a strong kink-informed referral network is crucial. Overall, being aware of the prevalence of sadomasochistic fantasies/desires, understanding and differentiating pro-social sadism from other typologies, and being able to navigate the distinctions between potentially beneficial BDSM play and potentially problematic sadistic or antisocial impulses require a high degree of discernment, careful documentation, and ongoing self-reflection by the clinician. Do not rush to pathologize your sensation-seeking clients; but be willing to do the hard work of risk assessment, safety planning, psychoeducation, and curious conversation in order to meet best the needs of both your kinky clients and your clinical practice.

ADDITIONAL RESOURCES

Perverse Psychology by Jemma Tosh

The Good Psychopath's Guide to Success: How to Use Your Inner Psychopath to Get the Most Out of Life by Dr. Kevin Dutton and Andy McNab

Sadomasochism: Powerful Pleasures by Peggy Kleinplatz and Charles Moser (eds.)

Screw the Roses, Send Me the Thorns: The Romance and Sexual Sorcery of Sadomasochism by Molly Devon and Phillip Miller

Hurts So Good: The Science and Culture of Pain on Purpose by Leigh Cowart

POWER EXCHANGE ROLEPLAY
Elyssa Helfer

IMAGINATIVE POWER EXCHANGE

There comes a point in the lives of most adults when imagination begins to dwindle; when the realities and responsibilities of life take hold and consume more and more space until the playful, adventurous, fantastical parts of ourselves are completely shut down. Without a consistent and intentional emphasis on play, the pursuit of play seems to fade from our consciousness, leaving only memories in its place. While routine, rigidity, seriousness, and stress may be at the forefront of the adult experience, many people have found a way to rewrite that script. There is one particular subset of the kink community where imagination is not only encouraged but celebrated; where the confines of age, gender, or even our species no longer matter, and we are free to lean into the expansiveness of our deepest fantasies. Imaginative power exchange is just that: a space where power exchange calls on imagination to roleplay an age different from our own, a taboo circumstance, an animal we wish to embody, and so much more.

> While the notion of playfulness intermeshes with those of exploration, curiosity and experimentation, it also foregrounds pleasure and bodily intensity as key motivations for sexual activity. Sexual play, driven by the quest for pleasure and the intensification of the body, probes and stretches the horizons of what people may imagine themselves as doing, liking and preferring. By doing so, it pushes sexual identifications into motions of varying speeds and lengths.
>
> Paasonen, 2018

DOI: 10.4324/9781003312833-5

CAREGIVER KINKS

One of the more widely misunderstood subcultures of kink exists at the intersection of imagination, playfulness, nurturance, and caregiving; these are the caregiver kinks. Due to the taboo nature of roleplay involving taking on a biological age different than one's actual age, the conflation of caregiver kinks and pedophilic disorder (see Chapter 8 for a thorough description of pedophilic disorder) is typical among those unfamiliar with the particular dynamics that accompany this kink. However, whether as a provider working with kinky folks, as someone who identifies as kinky, or as someone who is committed to pursuing and advocating for sexual freedoms, it is crucial that the differentiating factors between caregiver kinks and pedophilic disorder are not only acknowledged but deeply understood.

Age Play

While the literature regarding age play remains relatively limited, Paul Rulof—author of *Age Play: From Diapers to Diplomas* (2011)—provided an in-depth overview of age players, which has allowed researchers and kinksters alike to take a closer look at this intensely misunderstood group. As its name suggests, the subset of BDSM known as "age play" is a roleplay dynamic between consenting adults of legal age where at least one participant actively embodies or takes on the role of an age different than their biological age. One of the unique and often appealing facets of age play is that it does not follow any particular situational, relational, or social script, allowing participants to personify gender-diverse or heteronormative versions of the roles they seek to represent (Tiidenberg & Paasonen, 2019). The one area that does appear to be consistent among all age players is the pursuit of play:

> Approaching sexuality through the notion of play allows for crossing and bringing together of several notions often considered mutually exclusive, or at least positioned as being in persistent friction with one another. For if sex is understood as the stuff of adult experience, and not that of minors, then adults are excluded from the realm of play. Sexuality has often been considered as indicative of the end of both childhood and play (Bauer 2018, p. 145). Scholars have distinguished between childhood sexual play and adult activities by contrasting the former's "curiosity and playfulness" with the latter as "marked by an understanding of sexual behaviour and its consequences" (Essa & Murray, 1999, p. 232). Following

this line of thinking, play is innate to children and indicative of overall openness towards the world, yet something that ends and congeals as people age. In contrast, if one understands sexuality through the conceptual prism of play as acts of exploration motivated by pleasure within which different preferences and tastes are forged, no such categorical distinction needs to be made.

Tiidenberg & Paasonen, 2019

Contrary to the myth that all kink play involves sex, age play does not necessarily exist solely as a means for sexual connection and in many cases those who engage in age play do so without any play that is sexual in nature. That said, for some age players, sexual intimacy is one of the facets of their play. Upon reflection, the multiplicities of age-play identities, dynamics, and interactions highlight the colorful and expansive nature of age play; and attempting to utilize normative constructs to maintain a grasp of age play virtually erases the many complexities of these communities. "Encompassing diverse dynamics and rhythms, age-play involves the exploration of bodily capacities and desires that make it possible to move between different roles and thrills" (Tiidenberg & Paasonen, 2019). It is the fluidity of BDSM that makes it so profoundly freeing to experience yet challenging to comprehend.

The experiences that influence a kinky individual's desire to engage in age play are not universal. While it may be common to assume that age play is a maladaptive coping technique utilized to reprocess unwanted childhood experiences, it can be far more complex to understand—or in some cases, far more straightforward. For some, the draw to age play exists solely around its taboo nature. The concept of being simultaneously seduced and repulsed by something is not unprecedented. The thrill that accompanies even the thought of violating social norms—particularly in the case of sexual taboos—is exceptionally alluring and, further, not uncommon. Justin Lehmiller's research examining the sexual fantasies of over 4,000 participants found that "taboo and forbidden sex" ranked among the top five sexual fantasies (Lehmiller, 2018). Thus, it is unsurprising that there are folks whose age play is part of a sexual fetish (Rulof, 2011) or whose age-play experiences tend to be sexual in nature. Known among the kink community as "dark age play," this particular way of engaging in age play does involve sex and leans heavily into the taboo. To be an adult in a world full of constant chaos, stress, and an overabundance of responsibilities can and does overwhelm even the most regulated and composed individuals.

Many age players—particularly those who take on the role of "littles"—step out of the heaviness and burdensome nature of adult existence and lean into their childlike identities. While the definitions for "littles" can be slightly different depending on how folks are engaging with their age-play dynamics, to identify as a "little" means that someone is taking on the younger role within the relational space, which can range anywhere from roleplaying an infant all the way to embodying the identity of a teenager. Thus, an accurate definition of a "little" is someone who roleplays an age prior to the age of adulthood. That said, there are some folks whose "little" identities are not necessarily childlike and do not resonate with the title of "little." For these folks, the term "middle"—which commonly defines age players whose chosen role is typically one that is post-puberty (12–18 years)—may feel more accurate.

While "littles" and "middles" are a couple of identities held within the age-play community, their counterpart is typically considered the "caregiver"—which, unsurprisingly, is the person who adopts the role of caretaking, ranging anywhere from nurturing to authoritative. Due to the frequency of the parent/child relational roleplay, it is often assumed that the person in the caregiver role takes on either the "Mommy" or "Daddy" identity; however, far more identities can be embodied within an age-play dynamic. For example, a caregiver can take on the identity of a babysitter, teacher, doctor, and more. There is truly no particular configuration that must exist within an age-play dynamic, leaving room for varied and expansive relational formations. In fact, age play can be "a preference, an interest, a like, a point of identification, and anything beyond" (Tiidenberg & Paasonen, 2019). In addition, age play exists outside of the gender binary, opening the door to opportunities for roleplaying within a dynamic that allows for "renegotiating masculinity and femininity in relation to age, power and sexist stereotypes, as well as compensation for queer- and gender-related limitations experienced in one's own childhood" (Bauer, 2017).

There are a variety of identities and relational pairings that may be embodied by folks who engage in age play. However, it is important to note that the terms "Mommy" and "Daddy" are sometimes used outside of an age-play dynamic. In these cases, those terms are often utilized as a means to highlight the power hierarchy within the relational dynamic. They are not necessarily indicative of an age-play-based relationship. The following are some of the more commonly utilized relational pairings within the age-play community:

- **DDlg:** Daddy Dom little girl.
- **DDlb:** Daddy Dom little boy.
- **MDlg:** Mommy Dom little girl.
- **MDlb:** Mommy Dom little boy.
- **TDlb:** Trans Daddy little boy.
- **TDlg:** Trans Daddy little girl.
- **TMlb:** Trans Mommy little boy.
- **TMlg:** Trans Mommy little girl.
- **CGl:** Caregiver little.

As we have discussed, an unfortunate commonality among many adults is the complete disregard for play. Following our youth, the concept of play is no longer encouraged; nor is it intentionally integrated into one's life. When reflecting on the concept of play outside of a kink context, there seems to be a negative correlation between play and aging, meaning the older someone gets, the less they are engaging in some sort of play. Age play virtually overrides the unspoken notion that play does not belong in our adult lives and reignites the playfulness, wonder, and inclination toward adventure that steadily decline after entry into adulthood. In addition to age play being a vessel for the reintroduction of play, it can allow for the opportunity to rewrite or relive parts of childhood from a more controlled and intentional perspective. Perhaps there were strict rules in the home growing up; or specific clothing, toys, or experiences were not possible due to financial stressors. Age-playing as an adult can allow for childhood's unmet dreams or fantasies to finally become a reality.

We cannot talk about age play without noting the concept of regression: essentially, the idea that folks can revert to a psychologically younger state of mind. Regression within the age-play context is vastly understudied; however, it appears that regression accompanying age play is more so voluntary; whereas regression outside of a BDSM context can range anywhere from a voluntary attempt to alleviate stress to an involuntary psychological protective measure potentially indicative of a mental health condition (Simone, 2022). That said, there appear to be similarities between the experiences of "subspace" and the experiences of "little space," which calls into question the extent to which regression during age play is genuinely voluntary and further if regression during age play is even the correct way to describe the psychological experience of the "little" in general.

Fundamentally—and for many, most importantly—a common thread that ties most caregiver kinks together lies within the name itself, with the emphasis on care. Whether from the perspective of giving care (e.g., taking on the role of caretaker, Daddy, Mommy) or receiving care (e.g., taking on the role of little, middle), there is a reciprocal exchange of nurturance that permeates the various relational constellations that fall beneath the umbrella of caregiver kinks. One anonymous participant in Tiidenberg & Paasonen's research described just how important leaning into that care can be:

> "Today I just want to surrender. I want someone else to worry about the details, take care of this mouth and this body. I want someone else to make all of the choices and do all of the thinking. I want to succumb to caring hands, soothing sounds, full attention, good intentions. Let me be something precious."
>
> Tiidenberg & Paasonen, 2019

One of the most fundamental needs and desires of the human experience is the pursuit of love and belonging; and within an age-play dynamic, these needs can be and are met with guidance, tenderness, safety, support, and connection.

Adult Babies/Diaper Lovers

If you have never heard it before, "Don't yuck anybody's yum" is a phrase commonly used in many areas of life but it can be particularly valuable within the sex and kink world. This phrase—in the context of expressing and understanding BDSM interests—highlights the idea that while a sexual desire or behavior may not appeal to us personally, it is important to remain openminded and non-judgmental so that we do not contribute to emotional or psychological harm for the person whose interests are different than what is within our sexual repertoire or comfort level. This phrase is particularly important to keep in mind when learning about kink in general; however, it is even more vital as we move into discussing one of the most stigmatized subgroups of kinksters. As noted above, age players fall somewhere on a spectrum, ranging from babies to late teens. One of the most misunderstood and highly stigmatized subgroups within the kink community are those who identify with the youngest of the ages (infants/babies) or whose kink-related play requires diapers. These kinksters are referred to as "adult babies/diaper lovers" (ABDLs).

Similar to the other forms of age play described in the previous section, it is essential to emphasize that ABDL community members do not desire children; there is no attraction to children, nor are they interested in children in an inappropriate or non-consensual way. What they do desire can range from wanting to act, feel, or be treated like an infant to enjoying different sensations on their bodies to playing with the taboo nature of such a wide gap in their roleplay around age. Some "role-playing behaviors may include but are not limited to, using diapers, drinking out of a baby bottle, and a desire to be taken care of by a 'Mommy' or 'Daddy'" (Hawkinson & Zamboni, 2014). In addition, a number of other fetishes may also accompany ABDL roleplay, including urolagnia (urine fetish), coprophilia (feces fetish), and lactophilia (breast milk fetish) (Goerlich, 2023). One of the main contributing factors to the harsh criticism and discrimination that this community faces arises when folks are unable to separate the desire to be like a child from having a romantic or sexual interest in children.

An internet-based study of 1,795 male and 139 female self-identified members of the ABDL community concluded that there are at least two distinct subgroups within this community. These groups can be divided by their particular interest in influencing their community engagement. The researchers found that ABDL community members are interested primarily in either roleplay (adult babies) or sexual activity (diaper lovers) (Hawkinson & Zamboni, 2014). That said, diaper lovers may not be devoid of roleplay; nor are adult babies devoid of sexual engagement. Again, as with most kink identities, there is a fluidity within expression that may not fit perfectly into an internet definition.

Within the context of Hawkinson and Zamboni's research, they found that for diaper lovers, part of the sexual enjoyment was related to the perception that diapers were sexually stimulating and arousing. While for many, the sensation in and of itself is highly appealing, for others this type of engagement may play into humiliation and degradation. Where adult babies differed was that rather than diapers being particularly stimulating, other ABDL items (e.g., baby clothing, baby toys) appeared to be more appealing. In addition, if we zoom out and view this dynamic from a wider lens, there is evidence to suggest that "being dominated [is] an important part of ABDL behavior" (Hawkinson & Zamboni, 2014). This also applies to adult babies, whose roleplay enjoyment was similarly correlated with the perception of domination as a vital factor in ABDL behavior. Hawkinson and Zamboni suggested that "at a certain level, ABDL behavior may simply be a variant of sadomasochistic behavior in the sense that submissive or dominating behaviors are involved."

While limited research exists regarding this particular subset of the kink community, what appears clear is the severe impact of discrimination and stigmatization of ABDL community members. It is crucial to remain mindful of the diversity of sexual expressions and work to withhold judgment or assumptions when desires are different than one's own.

> Given the diversity of the ABDL community, clinicians and researchers should be cautious about making assumptions of persons involved in ABDL. Scholars should not assume that ABDL behavior is designed to cope with negative feelings. Given the general comfort and lack of distress with their ABDL behavior, future research might explore how persons involved with ABDL behavior became comfortable with their sexuality and how they made it work in their relationships.
>
> Hawkinson & Zamboni, 2014

While we live in a world where more than one thing can exist at once, to the point of Hawkinson and Zamboni, perhaps instead of focusing on the problems within "non-normative" communities and attempting to find something wrong, we can expand our minds and work on understanding why things might be going right.

PET PLAY

Roleplay takes on an entirely new form as we move out of the realm of human play and into the expansiveness of non-human play. Rather than embodying an age different from one's own or taking on a role intended to elicit the excitement of riding the edges of societal norms regarding sexual or relational connection, there are particular subsets of the kink community that push past the confines of human-to-human connection and inhabit non-human identities. Whether alone, with a partner, or in a group setting, pet players—with their varied features, identities, and social structures—lean into the imagination and, for many, reject the confines of human existence.

Assumptions about the pet play community are abundant—most notably those that conflate pet play with either zoophilia or bestiality, assuming that interest in pet play is indicative of an emotional or sexual attraction to animals. By definition, "zoophilia" is "a paraphilia in which nonhuman animals are repeatedly preferred or exclusively used to achieve sexual excitement and gratification" (APA Dictionary, 2023). "Bestiality" is "sexual excitement or gratification obtained by a human through . . . sexual contact with a nonhuman animal" (APA Dictionary, 2023). Pet play, as noted previously, does not involve animals; nor has there been research indicating that attraction, sexual or otherwise, to animals is present in pet players.

Another community often mistaken for pet players is the furry community. While furries are an additional subset of the greater kink community, rather than roleplaying an animal (e.g., a puppy, kitten, pony), furries are particularly interested in roleplaying anthropomorphic animals (e.g., mascots, Disney characters) (Hsu & Bailey, 2019). While there is an inherent power hierarchy within these relational dynamics (e.g., a handler and their pup), and these dynamics can certainly be a facet within an established D/s dynamic, it is always important to refrain from assumptions and allow pet players (and all kinksters, for that matter) to define how they identify themselves. Overall, pet play is a unique form of expression, heavily based on community, connection, and playfulness.

Pup Play

Pups are one of the most common subsets of the pet play community. "Pup/puppy play" is a form of roleplay in which consenting adults imitate and embody the behavior of dogs, primarily those which are young (puppies). Pup play may include sexual or erotic engagement or exist merely as a social activity; however, the motivating desires to participate in this type of play are incredibly expansive, allowing for different expressions of pup play depending on the context and setting (Wignall et al., 2022). For some, pup play is merely a social activity. For others, pup play is a way to express their innermost desires. While vastly understudied in formal research contexts, qualitative data collected from the pup play community and accounts of lived experience in various forums, blogs, and books have provided rich descriptions of what it means and what it looks like to be a pup.

When it comes to any form of kink expression, one of the primary questions that arises time and time again is simple: "Why"? The curiosity surrounding the "why" when it comes to sexual, erotic, or relational desire or engagement that is considered outside of the conventional norm seems to be addressed consistently. Attempting to fully understand why we might have a particular desire is a slippery slope; and in the case of kink, there is no evidence to suggest a single point of origin for these desires. What we do know is not necessarily *why* so many kinks have embedded themselves in the collective psyches of kinky folks, but *what* it is people enjoy about the kinks that encourages them to participate and engage.

In the case of pup play, for example, Langdridge and Lawson (2019) found that five themes came up regarding the desire to engage in pup play. The first theme that arose was the pursuit and enjoyment of sexual pleasure. Within various contexts, the experience of sexual pleasure is closely entwined with the dynamics of dominance and submission. Thus, taking on the role of pup/dog and being emotionally, relationally, and sexually subservient to a more dominant pup, handler, or other individual can be a motivating factor for engaging in pup play. In addition, they discovered that pup play allows for relaxation, feels like a form of therapy, and allows the kinksters to escape from self. In some cases, engaging in pup play can encourage individuals to shed the responsibilities that accompany adulthood, therefore allowing for a more carefree demeanor without societal narratives regarding "appropriate" adult behavior. On the contrary, the handler's role involves the responsibility of caring for their pups and is less about relaxation and more centered on elements of dominance, ownership, and care—particularly within D/s sexual dynamics. Pup play also encourages adult play and vibrant physicality. Being playful is one of the major draws to pup play, given the inherent physicality and active nature of many pup play activities—specifically "running around on all fours barring balls to and fro, playing rough and tumble with each other, or otherwise being 'playful puppies'" (Langdridge & Lawson, 2019). The researchers also saw the theme of extending and expressing selfhood. A psychological benefit of pup play appears to occur as handlers/pups can explore various dimensions of their personality. Someone who is typically shy may have the opportunity to lean into their confidence and playfulness. Pup play encourages growth and the chance to try on new aspects of one's identity. Lastly, and for some most importantly, pup play emphasizes relationships and community. The researchers found that many of those who engaged in pup play cultivated profound and significant connections with their peers, including other pups, packs, and handlers, as well as the local and global pup community.

Other Forms of Pet Play

In addition to pups and kittens, there are a number of other animals and creatures that may be embodied for pet players. For example, farm animals—such as ponies, pigs, cows, and other livestock—are common identities that are assumed while engaging in this type of play. Further, pet players may have an interest in roleplaying wild animals, including wolves, bunnies, and foxes. All types of pet play involve personalized dynamics that fit the roles of those participating; however, many of these relational dynamics are grounded in some sort of dominant/ submissive hierarchy. These may include aspects of degradation and humiliation (e.g., a pig being forced to urinate in the backyard) or utilization of elements, such as nature (e.g., a wolf chasing a fox through a forest). As with most other types of imaginative roleplay, these dynamics lean into creativity, fun, connection, and trust.

Roleplaying mythical creatures is yet another way to engage in pet play. Justin Lehmiller's (2018) research, as described in his book *Tell Me What You Want*, found that 33% of his participants had experienced sexual fantasies about a mythical creature. Lehmiller's work uncovered that gender and sexual orientation were differentiating factors for the kinds of mythical creatures that people found appealing. He found that among heterosexual women, 63% reported fantasizing about vampires, 9% fantasized about werewolves, and 8% fantasized about demons. At 26%, vampires were the highest category of fantasy for heterosexual men; however, 17% fantasized about demons, 12% about mermaids, 11% about nymphs, and 9% about elves. He found that the most common mythical creature fantasies were among self-identified gender non-binary folks, with 56% reporting overall fantasies regarding mythical creatures. As is apparent, the possibilities when it comes to roleplaying are truly endless and will likely continue to expand along with the introduction of new movies, books, video games, and television characters.

RISKS AND BENEFITS

Overall, when it comes to imaginative roleplay, the emotional, psychological, and relational benefits are abundant. From receiving or giving care to leaning into new adventures to embodying an identity that feels more aligned and engaged with the community, the joys of this type of play are felt by many. However, even as conversations about kink become more commonplace and a high percentage of the population engage in some sort of kink activity, imaginative role-play is still considered non-normative. As with any non-normative identity, there are risks of discrimination, stigmatization, and a general lack of understanding by partners, family, and peers. Thus, it is imperative to cover the topic of minority stress when discussing a subgroup as misunderstood and misrepresented as those who engage in age or pet play. The idea that "stigma, prejudice, and discrimination [have] created a hostile and stressful social environment that causes mental health problems" is the fundamental theory when understanding minority stress (Meyer, 2003). Engaging in a community that is highly stigmatized not only can impact an individual because of the direct experience of discrimination, but can create a persistent psychological state of fear around being "outed." The expectation of adverse reactions, internalized kinkphobia, and the need to conceal one's identity are all factors that can contribute to poor mental health outcomes. Adequate coping strategies and ample social support can undoubtedly be utilized to combat the impacts of minority stress; however, it is necessary to remain cognizant of the risks.

ADDITIONAL RESOURCES

How To Train Your Little: A DD/lg Guidebook, Volumes 1–3 by J.E. Earl and J. L. Lucky

Sex, Psychology and ABDLs by Dylan Lewis and Rosalie Bent

The Snufflington School of Online Roleplay and Basic Training for Owners and pups: An Instruction Manual and Guide by Aloysius Snufflington III

Pony Play with subMissAnn by subMissAnn

Ageplay: From Diapers to Diplomas by Paul Rulof

6

FETISHES
Stefani Goerlich

WHAT IS A FETISH?

At its most basic level, a "fetish" (also called a "paraphilia" in the clinical world) is simply a strong sexual attraction to or desire for an object or body part that is not typically sexualized. As with all kinks, fetishes are time and place specific. In America, for example, breasts are typically considered to be sexualized body parts. They are privately eroticized and publicly censored in ways that would be unthinkable to someone living in Berlin, Germany or among the Koma people of Nigeria. However, should someone report to their American or German clinician that they can only experience arousal or achieve orgasm when they are able to kiss, lick, and fondle their partner's armpit, this would pique curiosity, since the underarm is not a body part typically sexualized in either culture.

Fetishes are not limited to physical erogenous zones. Many fetishists experience a strong sexual desire for inanimate objects, various materials, or specific sensations. "People talk about having a 'fetish' for anything about which they are preoccupied, including nonsexual objects, activities, and ideas" (Fedoroff, 2020). The notion that an idea may be fetishized can be difficult to wrap one's head around until we consider the ways in which this practice is present in real life. For example, cuckolding (the practice of a husband watching his wife have sex with another man, often while being verbally or otherwise humiliated by the two) could be described as an idea fetish. It is rooted in the idea that the observer-husband is inferior to the other man and that the act of watching his wife being pleasured by

DOI: 10.4324/9781003312833-6

someone else is a humiliating commentary on his own inadequacy. This is a stark contrast to the feelings of erotic pleasure and compersion that may be experienced by a male swinger watching his wife make love to another man at a lifestyle event. It is the idea behind the cuckolding that makes the two experiences different, even when the behavior itself is indistinguishable.

Sometimes, ambiguity around the differences between idea fetishes and object fetishes can lead the clinician down a path of pathologization that may not be an accurate reflection of their client's erotic expression. Age play, which we discussed in Chapter 5, is often misunderstood as an expression of suppressed pedophilia, the sexual desire for prepubescent children. Outside observers who are unfamiliar with the concept of fetishized regression roleplay and the cathartic benefits it can have for its practitioners often leap to the assumption that age players are fetishizing actual children, even if their partners are legally adults. The difference between age play and pedophilia in this example is the nature of the fetishized attraction. Age players are aroused by the nurturing dynamic that role play can create. Pedophiles are aroused by children. As one DDlg fetishist puts it:

> a little just finds joy and pleasure in a dynamic in which they can shed their adult "skin" for a bit and be spoiled and taken care of . . . There's no part of us that doesn't understand we are two consenting adults having sex and a relationship . . . Daddy Dominants aren't attracted to children in the least.
>
> Earl & Lucky, 2018

- **Materials fetishes:**
  - Leather (dermatophilia)
  - Fur (doraphilia)
  - Latex/rubber
  - Silk/velvet (hypephilia)
  - Lace
  - Metal (metalliphilia)
  - Water (undinism)
  - Dirt/mud (molysmophilia)
  - Stone (lithophobia)
  - Wood (xylophilia)

- **Object fetishes:**
  - Statues/mannequins (agalmatophilia)
  - High heels (altocalciphilia)
  - Balloons
  - Thunder/lightning (keraunophilia)
  - Machines (mechanophilia)
  - Forests (nemophilia)
  - Snakes (ophidiophilia)
  - Dolls (pediophilia)
  - Fire (pyrophilia)
  - Trains (siderodromophilia)
- **Body fetishes**
  - Amputated limbs (acrotomophilia, amelotasis)
  - Pregnancy (cyesolagnia)
  - Tears, crying (dacryphilia)
  - Passing gas/farting (eprectolagnia, flatuphilia)
  - Foot fetishes (podophilia)
  - Blood (haematophilia) or menstruation (menophilia)
  - Lactation/breastfeeding (lacataphilia)
  - Shorter partners (nanophilia)
  - Teeth (odontophilia)
  - Stuttering, speech impediments (psellismophilia)
- **Behavioral fetishes:**
  - Financial exploitation (chrematistophilia)
  - Dirty talk, using obscenities (coprolalia)
  - Traveling (ecdemolagnia)
  - Sleeping (hypnophilia)
  - Tickling (knismolagnia)
  - Public speaking (laliophilia)
  - Watching one's partner have sex with someone else (mixoscopia, troilism)
  - Pretending to be dead (necrobiophilia, pseudonecrophilia)
  - Driving/riding in cars (amaxophilia)
  - Mocking/teasing (catagelophilia)
- **Idea fetishes:**
  - Being dirty/defiled (automysophilia, stercoracism) or dirtying/defiling others (salirophilia)
  - Dangerous/criminal partners (hybristophilia)
  - Sexual incompetence (harmatophilia)

- Failure (kakorrhaphiophilia)
- Novelty (neophilia)
- Sin, sinning (pecattiphilia)
- Poverty (peniaphilia)
- Being eaten/swallowed whole (voraphilia)
- Jealousy (zelophilia)
- Knowing that others are aware of your sexual behaviors (agrexophilia)

COMMON FETISHES

While both age play and armpit-licking can be startling to a clinician whose client is disclosing their desires for the first time, both practices are remarkably common. Very few studies have been done specifically on the prevalence of age play. However, this is a practice that has gained cultural traction in recent years, with its symbology and esthetics already represented within the mainstream. One team of researchers studying ABDL specifically (the most niche of age play dynamics) found "tens of thousands of videos, photos, and private blogs . . . all these data points indirectly to the fact that paraphilic infantilism is not limited to individual cases but is a more widespread phenomenon" (Oronowicz & Siwak, 2016). As these subcultures become accepted within the mainstream, their status as fetishes does not change (they still represent an attraction to something that is not typically sexualized); but their cultural identification as a kinky behavior fades away, like masturbation in the Victorian era. It can be difficult for clinicians—much less laypeople struggling with confusion and shame around their desires—to clearly understand what fetishes are "normal" (in this case, normative/common), which often leads to the conflating of normativity with problematicity. It is crucial to understand—and be able to convey to clients—that their desire being rare is not the same as their desire being unhealthy.

Our understanding of fetishism as a phenomenon is still evolving. Even simple questions such as prevalence have proven tricky to pin down, with some studies ranging from 0.8% (Abel & Osborn, 1992) to 18% (Scorolli et al., 2007) of the population reporting that they have at least one fetish. This is clearly too wide of a spread to be useful academically. Outside of academia, surveys by popular relationship websites have found that 54.3% of men and 46.2% of women report having both an interest in and participation with at least one fetish (Bedbible Research Center, 2023). What did these

112,000 respondents report being the most interested in? The ten most popular fetishes were:

- feet and foot-related objects;
- infidelity/cheating (cuckhold/cuckquean);
- voyeurism;
- age play;
- exhibitionism;
- *anime/hentai;*
- body fluids such as urine, feces, blood, or breast milk;
- body size (e.g., big, beautiful women);
- strength and musculature; and
- animal/pet play.

Ibid

HISTORY OF FETISHISM

When discussing fetishes and fetishistic disorders, we cannot separate our understanding of the psychology from our understanding of the social and cultural history. After all, the very term "fetish" has evolved from something that carried specific cultural and religious meaning to our modern concept of fetishes as primarily erotic in nature. Understanding how we got from Point A to Point B is crucial in understanding the extant confusion about the origins of sexual fetishes and fetishistic behaviors.

The creation and veneration of fetish objects is a near-universal cultural practice. In some cultures, this takes the form of totemic objects that symbolize specific qualities (e.g., fertility, strength, cunning, health) that are believed to be bestowed by god(s) upon the owner/wearer or their people (Learn, 2022). For others, the fetish might be a doll or puppet, created to look like a specific person or deity and believed to be energetically linked to the figure whose image it bears (Frankfurther, 2019). Even today, "modern" mainstream religious groups offer blessed objects to their followers to foster a sense of connection to their god. The notion that people can connect with a material object on a deep psychological level and ascribe layers of meaning and power to it is neither new nor particularly novel. It is, in many ways, a primal human behavior.

The term "fetish" was not originally a psychosexological term. Rather, it was coined in 1760 by Charles de Brosses in his work *On the Cult of the Fetish Gods.* As the study of other cultures developed as an academic discipline, European colonial observers coined the term "fetish" to describe cultural artifacts believed to have supernatural powers, serve as a connection between the human and the divine, or represent religious deities and concepts. "The critical characteristic of the religious fetish is that it derives its power from its associations with a deity" (Cumberpatch, 2000). These were often carved figures but could also include natural materials such as stones or feathers, or even collections of objects imbued with magical energy when the proper ceremonies were performed. Because of the cultural biases of these early observers, who assumed that their Western traditions were more rational and developed than those of the "primitive" others they studied, the notion of fetishes was imbued from the start with skepticism and bias. The creation and reverence of fetishes were viewed as irrational superstition rather than as a neutral, or even positive, cultural difference (Marie & Jordan, 2017).

As animism and tribal cultures were absorbed (or eradicated) by colonializing powers, practices that were simply long-held traditions became "different" enough from the newly modern social norms to merit curiosity from the emerging social science disciplines. Colonial notions of rationality and civilization certainly would have influenced Sigmund Freud's conceptualization of sexual fetishism. In this case, Freud proposed that fetish objects were defensive objects (not dissimilar in that respect to their early religious function), which allowed fetishists to protect themselves from sexual anxieties such as castration. Unlike the creators of some religious fetishes, however, Freud understood that sexual fetishists understood that their fetish was a symbolic, rather than literal protection.

> In his essay on "Fetishism," he wrote that "the fetishist is able *at one and the same time* to believe in his phantasy and to recognize that it is nothing by a phantasy. And yet, the fact of recognizing the phantasy *as phantasy* in no way reduced its power over the individual."
>
> Felluga, 2011

Freud's psychosexual perspective expanded the discourse around the nature and purpose of fetishes and brought the notion of adoration of the fetish object out of the realm of religion and culture and into the intimate domains of the mind and bedroom.

Freud's ideas were grounded in the work of Richard von Krafft-Ebing and Albert Moll, who had labored to move the conversation away from a religious framework of sin versus purity and toward a medical model. This was a crucial development because prior to the application of principles of medical health, sexually deviant people were typically classified as either sinners (who held aberrant desires but did not break the law) or criminals (those who committed rape, sodomy, or other sexual crimes). "Their main thrust was that in many cases, irregular sexual behavior should not be regarded as sin and crime but as symptoms of pathology" (Oosterhuis, 2012). The idea that differences in sexual expression and desire had physiological or psychological roots and therefore could be treated medically, as any other disease might be, was revolutionary. Indeed, in many ways, the world was not ready for this revolution. Much of the work of early sexologists (Freud, von Krafft-Ebing, Hirschfeld) was censored or destroyed completely in less than a century when the Nazis came to power.

It was not until the 1950s, when Albert Kinsey began his massive studies of male and female (heterosexual, cisgender, predominantly white) sexual behavior, that the scientific community began to discuss differences in sexual expression and erotic desire—and to understand their prevalence—in earnest. Since the introduction of Kinsey's work, sociologists, psychologists, sexologists, and physicians have generally accepted Freud's position that one's erotic map is not a moral failing. More recently, in the last 30 years, the mental health community has rejected elements of von Krafft-Ebing and Moll's medical model—most specifically, the notion that sexual deviance can be reduced or eliminated through medical treatment, a perspective that opened the door to horrific practices such as conversation and aversion therapies. This is not to say that biological theories for the etiology of fetishes have been completely ruled out. Rather, the rise of behavioral science (concurrent with, but not connected to, Kinsey's work) and our understanding of attachment theory have created a patchwork of "nature versus nurture" theories that each have both their proponents and detractors. Each offers its own explanation for which behaviors are "normal" versus "aberrant," which are rooted in biology and experience, which are mental illnesses, and which . . . simply *are*.

IS FETISHISM A MENTAL ILLNESS?

Until quite recently, much of the existing research focused on "extreme" examples of fetishism—those who have been hospitalized or incarcerated. These institutionalized subjects sometimes represented examples of fetishistic paraphilia (e.g., burglars whose primary target of theft was their fetish object; people with mental illness who struggled to self-regulate their desires in socially acceptable ways), making it difficult for researchers to parse out what constituted healthy/adaptive expressions of unconventional sexual desire from what was genuinely problematic for the individual and their community. As a result, many of the etiological theories regarding fetishism began from a place of assumptive disorder—that fetishes were born out of causes such as anxious or disrupted attachment to parents (Zamboni, 2017); trauma (Weisel-Barth, 2013); developmental disruptions (Abel et al., 2008); altered temporal lobe function (Masuda et al., 2014); or even substance misuse (Mehdizadeh-Zareanari et al., 2013). If it seems like these represent a relatively wide field of possible origin stories, that would be correct. There are two primary challenges in understanding where fetishes come from. The first is that there are too many different fetishes representing different forms of sensorimotor experience, emotional activation, relational dynamics, and behavioral patterns to ever be captured in a single Grand Unified Theory of Kink. The second problem is the issue of *time and place*. Fetishes are quite often so culturally specific that it can be a challenge for the global community of sexological researchers to reach a consensus even around what constitutes a fetish versus a normative erotic/sexual expression. The diagnosis of sexual paraphilias has been put forth as the solution to this cultural quandary by focusing not on the object itself (with a few notable exceptions), but rather on the intensity of the desire and the way this desire is enacted.

OBJECTOPHILIA

Objectophilia is a relatively rare manifestation of fetishism in which the object becomes not only a necessary component of the individual's erotic/arousal map but also the focus of a deep emotional or even romantic bond. Objectophiles form primary romantic attachments not to other people with whom they engage in fetish play but rather to the objects themselves (Kabiry, 2020). From cars to buildings to national landmarks and household appliances, objectophiles often believe that these objects have some form of consciousness or personality, will give their object a name or specific character traits, and may take these connections to the point of organizing a formal commitment ceremony to the (literal) object of their affection.

The term "objectophilia" was coined in the early 2000s and received a great deal of pop culture attention thanks to television documentaries such as *Married to the Eiffel Tower* and various reality programs. That said, objectophilia is not officially recognized by the mental health establishment as a psychiatric disorder or sexual orientation. This may be due to the objective rarity of objectophilia, which may be identified as a simple paraphilia or fetishistic disorder not otherwise specified during the assessment phase, and the propensity for objectophiles to exhibit co-occurring behaviors/concerns that are more likely to be formally assessed by their providers.

Attachment disorders and a history of trauma are not uncommon in self-identified objectophiles. Experiences of abuse, social phobia, and a history of rejection by other humans may lead objectophiles to take comfort in objects that cannot reject, hurt, or abandon them. Like other fetishists, some objectophiles may have had early experiences that created a strong attachment, or erotic imprint, to a particular object or type of object. It is also possible that objectophilia is correlated in some way with neurodivergency and autism spectrum disorder (Gatzia & Arnaud, 2022), but the research on this topic is scant. Some clinicians link objectophilia to obsessive-compulsive disorder and believe that these intense emotional attachments to inanimate objects serve as a form of coping strategy or, less charitably, a defense mechanism for those experiencing significant emotional difficulties.

The small sample size of objectophiles and the lack of research into this population have resulted in many theories but little evidence that can inform our understanding of this phenomenon. As with all unique sexual and relational diversities, we must approach clients who identify as objectophiles with respect, empathy, and openminded curiosity. Regardless of one's perspective, it is crucial to approach the topic with empathy and respect for the individuals involved while also considering the ethical implications related to consent and boundaries.

DIGISEXUALITY

Digisexuality, robosexuality, and teledildonics are related but distinct erotic desires/fetishes that fall under the umbrella of "technosexuality"—that is, any practice involving the eroticization of technology. Dr. Trudy Barber, who coined the term in 2005, observed that members of sexual subcultures were early adopters of new technologies. Her research into the ways in which fetishists particularly interacted with technology made her one of the first to recognize the role that emerging technologies played in shifting how humans enact intimacy together and understand themselves as sexual beings:

> Fetishists . . . appear to engage creatively with new technology, rather than ignoring it or being fearful and misunderstanding it. Fetishists will try to subvert, modify and adapt new technologies to suit their own predilections. It is the unanticipated adaptation of technology through fetishism that may be central to creating new designs for future use of technologies that will permit new possibilities of pleasure, leisure and entertainment, intimacy, innovative interaction and arousal. This possibility has already contributed to unexpected and unforeseen forms of sexual behavior . . . and will make us re-assess our possible consumption of pleasure and leisure and to consider, for example, the consequences for the entertainment industry, sexual health, forensic sexology, issues of morality and the law.
>
> Barber, 2004

Digisexuality, teledildonics, and robosexuality are some of the "new possibilities of pleasure" that Barber foresaw. "Digisexuality"—a term coined by Drs. Markie Twist and Neil McArthur in 2017—refers to people who find interactions with technology such as virtual reality (VR) or artificial intelligence (AI) integral to their sexuality, to the point where they may prefer erotic interactions with technology over sexual interactions with humans. Our understanding of digisexuality as a practice and potentially as an identity is still emerging; and (much like with other BDSM/kink practices) it may be understood as a form of recreation, a lifestyle, or an orientation by different clients at different times.

> We draw a distinction between digisexualities, the technologies that allow for sexual experiences, and what we call digisexuals, people who see themselves as possessing a distinctive form of sexual identity. We can think of the distinction between those who mere use digisexual technologies on the one hand, and digisexuals as an identity-group on the other, according to analogies with other sexuality-based identities . . . Many people engage in kinky, non-monogamous, or same-sex behavior, but only a certain percentage of such people actually link their sexual identity to this behavior. Thus, we can imagine a future . . . where people identify along a digisexual continuum, with those at an extreme end considering digisexualities as an integral part of their sexual identity and not as a mere fetish or kink.
>
> McArthur & Twist, 2017

Scan to see a short
documentary about
HarmonyX, one of the
most technologically
advanced robot
companions on the
market today.

Figure 6.1   Short HarmonyX Documentary (QR code)

For some, this is already happening. "Teledildonics," a term first coined in 1977 by hacker Ted Nelson to describe computer network-facilitated sexual expression, has existed for as long as we have had modern technology. The telegraph, for example, was used to wire "sexts" across the country; and as soon as the telephone was invented, so was phone sex (Goerlich, 2022). Today, partners on opposite sides of the world can experience synchronized erotic sensations via paired, app-controlled, Bluetooth-enabled sex toys. In addition to the plethora of high-tech devices enabling one to stay sexually connected to one's partner from a distance, there are also new technologies that allow people without human partners to experience erotic connections as well. Sex dolls made by companies such as Real Doll (which also owns robotics company Realbotix) use AI and thousands of tiny motors to create hyperrealistic machines that are capable of responding not only physiologically (e.g., warming to the touch, lubricating genitals), but conversationally as well. Robosexuals, a subculture within the digisexual community, prefer these robotic partners to humans—which can be difficult considering the high cost of these machines and the ongoing stigma experienced by those who own/use them.

Rather than spending upwards of $7,500 on a robotic sex doll, many digisexuals turn to VR and AI.

> Research indicated that intimacy and passion, which are reflected by strong emotional connections and passionate feelings, can be forged between humans and objects as between human beings . . . For intelligent assistants, which are highly anthropomorphized, it is most likely that users may generate emotional connection and passionate feelings for them in some contexts.
>
> Song et al., 2022

Apps such as Replika and Character.ai allow users to create an AI personality that responds to them as if it were a human partner—with humor, flirtation, support, and eroticism. This is not to say that everyone who creates an AI partner does so because they do not have real relationships. Many users are engaging erotically with AI in addition to maintaining their human relationships. As with other object fetishes, depending upon the negotiated relationship agreements and the degree of transparency, this may or may not be perceived as cheating by either the user or their human partner (Nolan, 2023).

RISKS AND BENEFITS

It is difficult to give a definitive answer regarding the risks and benefits of object fetishism because so much depends upon the specific fetish and the specific client. We know from the literature that the vast majority of object fetishists are mentally and emotionally healthy people who engage in private erotic expression that simply falls outside of what is considered "normally sexual" for their time and place. Risk assessment, then, is a highly personalized process that must take into account the nature of the fetish object (e.g., knee socks carry less risk of harm than knives) and the actions of the client in relation to the fetish object. Someone who has a knee sock fetish is not necessarily at risk of harm—until or unless their desire for knee socks leads them to begin stealing socks from stores, fondling the legs of nonconsenting sock wearers, or otherwise bringing the benign fetish object into a more problematic behavioral pattern—often appearing alongside concerns such as hypersexuality or other non-object paraphilias (Eusei & Delcea, 2020). In the absence of problematic or compulsive behaviors related to the object fetish, the clinician should err on the side of affirming the client's attraction and helping them process any feelings of guilt or shame that may arise due to their desires. After all, "Separating sexual behaviors (paraphilias) from the mental disorders (paraphilic disorders) is the first step in depathologizing consensual alternative sex" (Wright, 2010).

Scan to listen to Securing Sexuality, a weekly podcast about the intersections of intimacy and technology.

Figure 6.2 The *Securing Sexuality* Podcast (QR code)

The risk/benefit conversation around the rise of digisexuality is more nuanced because this is a practice that is developing concurrently with technology as it advances and thus has not been studied in any longitudinal way. This leaves us with a growing population of clients engaging with newly emerging technologies and inadequate information regarding the long-term outcomes of their use. The rapid evolution of technology makes conducting this research nearly impossible because by the time we have sufficient data to draw conclusions, the tools we are studying have faded from popular use. For example, it would not be useful to study the relationship outcomes of cybersex website users in the 1990s and try to apply these to AI chat app users today. Researchers and ethicists have proposed many potential benefits for greater use of AI, ranging from workplace assistants and research tools to virtual caregivers and mental health providers, to name just a few. As our use of AI increases and becomes normalized, our clients will humanize these tools and form relationships with them as caregivers and friends, partners, and lovers; and we do not yet know how this will impact the individual mind or human relationships (Alegre, 2018). As with all emerging issues within psychology and sexology, the field is sorting itself into those who are proponents of technosexuality (Levy, HarperCollins), and those who advocate for restraint or even prohibition (Richardson, 2015). The kink-affirming clinician must undertake the often-difficult work of continuing education—even when the topic seems far afield from traditional mental health practice—and cultivating their own understanding of the ethical questions, potential risks, and suggested benefits of intimate technologies so that they can then provide the psychoeducational support their clients need.

ADDITIONAL RESOURCES

The Pleasure's All Mine: A History of Perverse Sex by Julie Peakman
Fetish: Fashion, Sex, & Power by Valerie Steele
Fantasies of Fetishism: From Decadence to the Post-Human by Amanda Fernbach
Female Fetishism: A New Look by Lorraine Gamman and Merja Makinen
Robot Sex: Social and Ethical Implications by John Danaher and Neil McArthur (eds.)

7

WHAT DOES A KINKY SCENE LOOK LIKE?

Elyssa Helfer

THE KINK COMMUNITY

Munches and Sloshes

The many inaccurate depictions of kinky folks in popular media have undoubtedly shaped the image of the kink persona. The brooding sadist; the broken and lost submissive; the dominatrix who almost always ends up being the villain on crime shows: these stereotypical tropes impede the public's ability to see kinksters for who they are; rather, they focus exclusively on what they do. When I ask you to imagine a gathering of kinky people, what comes immediately to mind? Perhaps you envision a dungeon space in which everyone has donned their favorite leather gear; or maybe the vision is a lust-fueled play party or a sexual free-for-all. If you have only the media's portrayals of kink as an example of kinky life, you may not have visualized a group of kinksters at a bowling alley or grabbing brunch at a local spot. Sometimes, folks can forget that kink involvement within the community can be just as important as it is within one's personal dynamic.

Social engagement is an integral part of the lives of kinky folks as, for many, the connections, guidance, and room for acceptance and understanding are vital in maintaining a healthy kink practice. Overall, community gatherings within the kink community "are based on interaction and ritual practices in social contexts including

DOI: 10.4324/9781003312833-7

clubs, private parties, pub evenings or workshops, where practitioners meet to socialize, learn and practice BDSM" (Carlstrom, 2018). So, while some kink gatherings do include some sort of play that is erotic or sexual in nature, there are various ways in which kinksters connect socially that can be just as—or even more—fulfilling.

Reportedly evolving from non-play social gatherings held in California in the 1980s (Weiss, 2006), "munches" have grown to become a central point of connection within the BDSM community, particularly for newcomers. Munches are social gatherings, typically in a public space, where no kink activities take place. For a community where there is a significant emphasis on personal, erotic, and sexual adventure and exploration, it can be exceptionally appealing to attend a low-pressure, informal, and play-free event where the focus is solely on community and connection building. It is helpful to note that the term "munch" is more often used internationally; while the term "slosh" is commonplace in North America, particularly the Midwest. While some folks use the terms "munch" and "slosh" interchangeably, one of the primary differentiating factors is whether the event centers around alcohol. Thus, munches tend to occur at restaurants or places where folks can munch (see what they did there?), while sloshes often occur at bars or pubs. Overall, these informal kink events serve as a conduit for newcomers as they begin to integrate into the BDSM community and exist as a staple for those who have already found a community of their own. In fact, in a recent survey of over 1,000 Fetlife users, about 68% of participants stated that munches are paramount to the kink experience, and about 65% reported that they attend a munch at least once per month. (Webster & Klaserner, 2019). While attending munches can undoubtedly serve as an excellent way to meet community members, there are a number of reasons why munches may not be the right fit for everyone in the community, including a lack of interest in being outed, difficulties related to location or simply lack of interest or investment in the community at large. However, for those who are interested in attending munches, they are most commonly discovered through Fetlife event pages, word of mouth, social media pages and Listservs.

Educational Events

If you have ever wondered why it can be such a struggle to research kink-related topics, you are not alone. Competing definitions of "kink" are one of the many reasons why it can be challenging to pursue kink research in an academic setting (alongside a lack of funding, minimal participant engagement, and more). While folks can undoubtedly settle on a way in which they define "kink," we cannot overlook the reality that kink, in many cases, is subjective. What one person considers outside of the conventional norm will not apply to everyone, and this shifting definition makes it difficult to distinguish what is truly considered kink and what is considered vanilla (or non-kink). Further, even when coming to a consensus on an operational definition of kink, a simple definition cannot fully encompass the nuance and complexities that arise when engaging in kink. Questions such as, "Is kink an identity or a hobby?" "Is kink a relational style?" and "Is kink a skillset?" are frequently discussed among kink researchers and kink participants alike—it may not come as a surprise to you, but often kink researchers are also kink participants. As for these questions, the answers are yes and no. Kink does not exist in a bubble and what is kinky to one person may not be kinky to another. Carlstrom noted that:

> it should be stressed that a minority, or a self-defined group such as a BDSM community, does not constitute a fixed identity. It can be reformed, and the community can jointly create new ideas about what identity is and should contain at a given moment.
>
> Carlstrom 2019

For this reason, it is vital to invest in kink education (and I do not necessarily mean financially), both if you are kinky and if you are someone who knows, loves, or works with or for kinky people. As an ever-evolving form of relational connection and expression, a helpful way to remain aware of these continuous changes is to pursue ongoing education.

To participate in kink responsibly means not only to assess one's level of experience as a participant in the community in general; vitally, if one attempts any form of engagement, that requires a skill. This is even more pressing when that skill involves the participation of someone aside from oneself. Whether learning how to use a flogger (a multi-tailed whip), a cane, a paddle, or even spanking, it is crucial to be mindful of the steps involved in engaging in a risk-aware, safety-focused way. Fortunately, educational opportunities are abundant in the kink community—that is, if you know where to look. Through mentorship, coursework, webinars, and more, gaining this knowledge is possible as long as the commitment to the craft is present. Remember, like many other activities, we cannot claim that kink is *always* safe. This is why education and risk awareness are crucial!

Local Educational Opportunities

Should kinky folks reside in an area that houses a local dungeon, they may have the opportunity to participate in educational opportunities in person. In addition to serving as a local play space and community center, many dungeons provide education to community members. Whether a BDSM 101 course or a *shibari* (Japanese rope tying) demo, a variety of topics can be covered, depending on the availability of community educators. Typically, kink-related workshops fall into two categories: educational (focused on disseminating information) and demonstration (focused on teaching or presenting a particular skillset). If you are wondering where your city's dungeon is or if it even has one, there are a few ways to find out. First, in highly populated cities, a Google search can bring up dungeon information. If simply searching the internet does not garner results, FetLife—the largest kink social media site—has an events tab that lists local events. Another very useful resource is word of mouth. If you find yourself attending a munch or community event, there may be an opportunity to learn more about what groups and organizations exist locally by inquiring among other community members.

Research/Educational Organizations

For those interested in pursuing kink education from an academic or professional lens, there are several kink research/educational organizations whose work centers the kink experience. While there are many programs offering kink-related education, the following are institutions whose sole focus is kink research, education, and advocacy:

- **The Alternative Sexualities Health Research Alliance★ (TASHRA)**: This is an organization whose "focus is on health disparities; injuries and medical complications from engaging in fetish, kink and BDSM activities; and the discrimination experienced in healthcare settings" (TASHRA, 2024). As a leader in the kink research world, TASHRA conducts "groundbreaking research and provide[s] cutting edge clinical training" with the goal of enhancing "the physical and mental health of people who engage in BDSM, kink and fetish practices." For more information, check out Tashra.org.
- **The National Coalition for Sexual Freedom★ (NCSF)**: This is a "nonprofit membership organization that advocates for

Figure 7.1 The Alternative Sexualities Health Research Alliance (TASHRA) (QR code)

Figure 7.2 The National Coalition for Sexual Freedom (NCSF) (QR code)

consenting adults in the kink and non-monogamy lifestyles by fighting discrimination and persecution through direct services." It provides "education for professionals about consent and the Alt-sex communities, including Continuing Legal Education for attorneys and Continuing Education Units for mental health professionals," as well as "for members of the BDSM-Leather-Fetish, Swing and Polyamory communities about consent and legal issues that may affect them." Lastly, it supports "the outreach and education efforts of groups, clubs and events to local law

Scan to view the website of the Science of BDSM research laboratory.

Figure 7.3   The Science of BDSM Lab (QR code)

enforcement, service agencies and authorities." (NCSF, 2024). For more information, check out NCSFreedom.org.

- **Science of BDSM:** "The Science of BDSM Research Team is led by professor of social psychology Dr. Brad Sagarin, composed of academics and community members. Members of the team include graduate and undergraduate students in a variety of fields, professors of psychology, clinical psychologists, and kinky people who are interested in supporting research. The team aspires to produce and disseminate quality research on BDSM (bondage/discipline,dominance/submission,sadism/masochism), and kink-related topics," as well as "to understand the nature, dynamics, motivations, and effects of BDSM activities and relationships" (Science of BDSM, 2024). For more information, check out ScienceofBDSM.com

- **Community-Academic Consortium for Research on Alternative Sexualities (CARAS)**: This "is a national-level, 501(c)(3) nonprofit organization that supports research addressing understudied sexualities, with a current focus on kink/BDSM/ leather/fetish sexualities, related sex work, and consensual non-monogamous relationships such as polyamory. Employing a community-based research model, CARAS has assembled a network of academics, clinicians and respected members of these communities who will work directly with researchers to promote scientific and other forms of scholarly research" (CARAS, 2024). For more information, check out carasresearch.org.

Scan to view the website of the Community Academic Consortium for Research on Alternative Sexualities.

Figure 7.4   The Community-Academic Consortium for Research on Alternative Sexualities (CARAS) (QR code)

The following is a non-exhaustive list of organizations that provide kink-related educational opportunities; however, they are not solely focused on kink education, but rather sex education as a whole:

- **Sexual Health Alliance** (https://sexualhealthalliance.com/)
- **Modern Sex Therapy Institutes**★ (modernsextherapyinstitutes. com)
- **The Beuhler Institute** (www.learnsextherapy.com/)
- **The Affirmative Couch**★ (https://affirmativecouch.com/)

★ A star denotes the author's professional affiliation with an organization.

Virtual Opportunities

Amid the heartbreak and isolation that accompanied the Covid-19 pandemic, a new way of engaging virtually opened the door to a host of online educational opportunities. In order to protect the health and safety of the kink community, many dungeons began providing workshops and educational events online. Creatively using the resources available, kinky folks began to engage with one another in virtual spaces where intentions were not only on connection but on education. From lectures to virtual demonstrations, a new world opened up, expanding the resource pool for people who may not have had access previously. Currently, online kink education remains abundant.

Whether someone is seeking coursework in a professional setting or a community setting, utilizing the internet for kink education is an excellent option for folks who may be geographically or physically unable to attend events and workshops in person. Lastly, and very importantly, virtual opportunities may be a great source of education for folks who do not have the means to invest financially in attending in-person events. If you already participate in BDSM, it will come as no surprise to you that participating in kink can be expensive:

> Access to BDSM spaces often requires a significant investment of economic resources—a fee for a membership to a dungeon (BDSM social club, educational venue, and play setting), an entrance fee for each event one attends, appropriate clothing (leather, latex, and other fetish gear), BDSM implements, and a host of related expenses.
>
> Graham et al, 2015

Attending virtual workshops may make the investment significantly smaller, if not free!

Online Communities

Suzanne van der Beek and Laura Thomas (2023) describe "social cohesion" as "an important dimension of the kink community," elaborating that "an important part of [that] cohesion is shaped via online platforms." They further explain that online kink platforms allow kinksters to "find each other and organize (offline) events such as munches (informal gatherings for anyone interested in kink), play parties (social events that facilitate kink play), and rope jams (meetings during which kinksters can practice rope techniques)" (van der Beek & Thomas, 2023). Fortunately, there are several socio-sexual networking sites that kinky folks can utilize (Zambelli, 2017), which have shifted away from the older kink subcultures that were predominantly organized around community venues (Steinmetz & Maginn, 2014; Wignall et al., 2022).

With the expansion of online kink communities and the ability to connect globally via the internet, a new generation have had the opportunity to explore and expand their kink interests (Zambelli, 2017). However, despite the relative ease that has accompanied this expanded access, a growing community means that previously established community norms may be questioned or altered. As new generations enter the kink community, they bring with them new ways of relating and, in some cases, a disregard for the spoken or unspoken standards of particular kink subcultures. For some communities, there seems to be a tug of war between folks who adhere to Old Guard principles, high protocol, sophisticated rules and etiquette; and The Next Generation, whose approach to kink is more lax, low protocol, and flexible. While many kink scholars feel that there is no "right" way to participate in kink as long as it remains consensual and between adults, there are folks who adamantly disagree—which, fortunately, allows for new generations of kinksters to decide which type of community they would like to access and potentially gain membership into. Online communities have opened the door to a flood of new approaches, rules, boundaries, and ways of engaging in kink—further contributing to the debate about what kink even is in the first place. What remains clear is that kink is an ever-evolving way of connecting with oneself, one another, and the world around us.

Finally, it is important to remember that while kink education is available from numerous different sources—from community members to researchers, academics, and more—just because someone is providing kink education does not necessarily mean that the education is right for you. Please vet organizations and educators prior to taking courses from them. You can do this by learning about their community engagement, checking their credentials, and trusting your instincts.

WHAT IS A "SCENE"?

One of the unique differentiating factors between BDSM engagement and what is considered "normative" vanilla sex is the intentionality that goes into envisioning, negotiating, executing, recovering from, and finally debriefing upon completion of a BDSM scene. In the context of kink, a "scene" is a pre-negotiated, consensual activity, engagement, or interaction that occurs between all participating parties. A "scene"—also referred to as a "session"—is the execution of the negotiated event and, perhaps most importantly, is sandwiched between a variety of vital steps that help folks prepare for and recover from the scene itself. Unlike vanilla sex, where a version of intercourse may occur more spontaneously, kink scenes are meticulously and intentionally planned, with an emphasis on consent, safety, acknowledgment of risk, and shared goals. This is not to say that kink scenes cannot have components of spontaneity within them; they are simply approached from a different perspective:

When these kinds of scenes do occur, they occur as sites of spontaneous interaction within a general set of rules. In this regard, they are more akin to improvisational theater than scripted performance. In improv, performers (who call themselves "players") create, and they often do not know what the scene will involve or where it will "take" them. The success of an improv scene depends in part on the "agreement" of the players, generally before the scene. This "likemindedness" refers not to the procession of a particular plot or the development of particular characters but a willingness to follow one another for the sake of the scene (Seham 2001). SM participants enter into play from a similar perspective; negotiation and consent set the parameters for a scene, and participants regard their interactions within those constraints as spontaneous, pure, and authentic.

Newmahr, 2010

In contrast to the common misconceptions around kink play, many BDSM scenes are non-sexual and may in fact involve a complete lack of physical touch. However, whether or not physical touch is involved, what is arguably even more important than the scene itself are the interactions that occur beforehand and afterward. When a BDSM-related fantasy arises, a number of steps can occur between the conception of the scene and the scene itself. Negotiation is one of the primary factors to increase the likelihood (not guarantee—as we cannot account for or predict all possible outcomes) of a self-defined successful scene. For some, a negotiation can occur relatively quickly, touching on the important points and ensuring that the main bases are covered. However, for others (particularly when exploring edge play), it can take weeks or even months to organize and solidify the scene and the following events.

NEGOTIATION

Negotiation is a concept many of us are intimately familiar with. As a child, we may have negotiated our bedtime or for an extra scoop of ice cream; as a teen, we may have attempted to negotiate a curfew; and as an adult, we may have negotiated our salary or pay. Fundamentally, negotiation is commonplace in our day-to-day experience and is typically done in order for all parties involved to reach an agreed decision about how an experience, event, or engagement will go—particularly when stakes are high. Wanting more candy as a child will not have the same impact or consequence as ensuring our pay is enough to keep food on the table. Thus, as we consider the potential risks that accompany BDSM play, the importance of negotiation becomes clearer.

Negotiation will look different from person to person and must be adapted to accommodate different communication styles, abilities, and comfort levels. It can occur at a single meeting or take place over the course of days or weeks. The "how" of negotiations (e.g., are checklists helpful or overwhelming? Should there be a written contract?) will depend on what works best for the parties involved; however, the "what" of negotiations is rather more standard. In order to be fully informed, there are several concepts to cover, each of which helps create a truly risk-informed, safety-prioritized, pleasure-focused experience.

The following concepts can be utilized to thoroughly prepare for a scene. There is no particular order to follow and some questions may not be appropriate given the type of scene; however, as for that child wanting that extra scoop of ice cream, the more, the better.

Goals/Intentions

BDSM scenes do not just happen without intent; something is fueling them and there is some outcome that folks are trying to achieve. It could be as simple as having a good time or as complex as properly executing a new skill. BDSM scenes have a purpose and it is important to discuss what that purpose is. Folks who are engaging in BDSM should discuss what the goals for the scene are, emphasizing what they are hoping to experience or achieve. Communicating and expressing shared goals not only makes the play more intentional, but also helps guide the direction of the play so that those goals are met.

Potential questions could include the following:

- What is the goal/intention for this particular scene?
- Are there any specific emotional/physical feelings that one or more participants are hoping for?
- Is this scene meant to induce feelings of sensuality? Playfulness? Catharsis? Helplessness? Etc.
- Is intercourse/orgasm a priority if the scene involves sexual contact?

Intensity

The scene's intensity can refer to many things; however, this is particularly important when any sort of pain or sensation is involved. Prior to beginning the scene, the intensity level must be negotiated

Figure 7.5   Kink and Scene Negotiation (QR code)

and agreed upon. For example, suppose a beginner is interested in impact play. In that case, they may agree that spanking at a medium-intensity level is comfortable, but they are willing to work toward a medium-high level of intensity. As "intensity" is an entirely subjective experience, there must be a way to indicate a medium intensity level. Using a number system (0–10) or a traffic-light system (red, yellow, green) can help assess the way in which someone relates to intensity. This part of the negotiation is particularly important when it comes to the concept of obtaining explicit prior permission (see Chapter 10 for a thorough explanation).

Potential questions could include the following:

- **Top:** How will I know that you are reaching your threshold for the level of intensity?
- **Bottom:** What is a clear way that I can indicate to you when I am nearing my threshold for intensity?

Limits

Limits can be divided into two primary categories: hard limits and soft limits. Hard limits are activities that are considered hard nos, which a party has no intention of ever participating in or pursuing under any circumstance. When a hard limit is set, it is crucial not to pressure, shame, or guilt someone into engaging in the relevant activity. Respecting limits is critical in negotiating a BDSM scene;

but while hard limits create a clear line between what is and is not welcome, soft limits are a bit more fluid. Soft limits fall within the maybe category, notably existing as activities that are not of particular interest, but that may be something an individual is willing to try should the circumstances, setting, and situation align. Limits help establish boundaries regarding what is and what is not acceptable during a scene.

A checklist may come in handy when it comes to hard and soft limits. Not only are there more types of kink engagement than one person can likely remember, but there are also new types of play arising frequently. Please follow the QR code for kink and scene negotiation checklists and worksheets.

Potential questions could include the following:

- What kink activities are you not willing to engage in?
- Are there activities that you might be willing to try?
- Are there soft limits you want to bring into play during this scene?
- If you notice something is a hard limit, but you have not realized it before, how will you indicate that to me during the play?

Safe Words/Gestures

An essential part of negotiating a scene is coming up with and disclosing safe words/gestures. A "safe word" is a pre-negotiated and clear signal that an activity must come to a complete stop. Due to the inherently risky nature of some BDSM activities and the many unpredictable human responses that can arise when engaging with new or intense stimuli, a safe word must exist so that no participants—regardless of identity or role—are pushed beyond their pre-negotiated or unexpected limits. In addition to a safe word, a safe gesture is an important signal to include in a negotiation. There are a variety of circumstances in which the ability to speak is not possible during a kink scene. In those cases, coming up with a gesture (e.g., tapping three times, snapping fingers) is crucial.

Tips for safe words include the following:

- Do not use words that are too complicated to remember mid-scene. (The traffic-light system is prevalent among kinksters:

red = stop; green = continue; yellow = remain cautious not to push much further).
- Ensure that safe words are consistent throughout play.
- Practice using safe words outside of the kink space.
- Always ensure that there are gestures put in place for moments when verbalizing is not possible.
- Do not choose a safe word that can be a part of the play (e.g., "no," "stop," "don't").

Physical Touch

As noted previously, BDSM does not always include sex; nor must it include any sort of physical touch. The use of touch must be negotiated, as well as what type of touch and where it is permitted. In terms of sexual touch, this is another area where it needs to be clearly defined prior to any engagement.

Potential questions could include the following:

- Is touch permitted in this scene?
- What parts of the body are okay to touch?
- What parts of the body are not okay to touch?
- In which ways do you prefer to touch/be touched?
- Is sexual contact permitted in this scene?
- Which types of sexual contact are welcome and which are off limits (e.g., anal/vaginal/oral penetration; anal/vaginal/oral stimulation)?
- Which methods of contact are welcome, and which are off limits (e.g., toys; fingers; tongue; genitals; all; none)?
- How will we ensure we remain cognizant of safety when including physical touch?

Scene Details

It may seem obvious, but it is important to negotiate the specific details of the scene. The details of the scene include negotiating the time, day, location, and all other details that may pertain to the scene. This can also include the use of toys, tools, instruments, or accessories that may be used. By discussing these details in advance, there will be no surprises (unless surprises are a part of the scene—which, again, should be negotiated!)

Potential questions could include the following:

- Where will the scene take place?
- How will we get to/from the scene?
- How long will the scene last for? How much time is planned for aftercare?
- Will other people be present for the scene?
- Will kink instruments be involved? Who is responsible for bringing them? How will the instruments be handled? What is your experience level using these particular instruments?
- In the case of sex toys, is it necessary that they are brand new/unused? If not, how will you ensure they are sanitary?

Risks

Risk is one of the items for negotiation that will likely take the most time. It covers various topics and, frankly, is one of the least fun or sexy parts of the negotiation. That said, it is one of the most important and should under no circumstances be skipped or overlooked. Risks can include everything from physical risks and health risks to emotional risks and even risks related to legal action/consequences. Physical/health risks are extremely important to discuss prior to any kink scene. If any health/medical risks could put a participant in danger, it is vital that all parties know not only what those risks are but what to do if one becomes a reality. Pertaining to legal risk, a concern that can easily be overlooked is how the setting of a scene may put participants at risk. An example of this is when a scene occurs within one's home and a nearby neighbor/roommate/person overhears. Folks who are unfamiliar with the kink engagement of those in a nearby space may hear what they believe is a person in danger and act accordingly. This is why it is vital to consider the environment in which someone is playing in addition to the play itself. Remember, just because the participants in the scene have consented does not mean that those in the general vicinity have consented as well. Emotional risks will be covered within the trigger plan category.

Potential questions could include the following:

- Are there any health/medical conditions that certain types of play may activate?
- Are there any allergies that can be activated during a scene (e.g., asthma, latex, leather)?

- Should a medical concern arise, what are the next steps (e.g., call an ambulance/a doctor)?
- What tools are necessary to ensure all participants remain safe (e.g., if rope is involved, will safety shears be nearby)?
- Is it possible that someone outside of the space may be able to hear or see the scene?
- How can we ensure that we will have privacy?

Marks

Many forms of BDSM play include activities that can leave marks on the body—most notably bruises, scratches, and cuts. While many kinksters view marks as a source of pride, wanting to show off the art created on their bodies, others may be adamantly against any visual evidence of their kink play. In addition to specifying physical touch on/off limit zones, inquiring about if and where marks may be left on the body is crucial.

Potential questions could include the following:

- Are you comfortable being marked?
- If so, which types of marks do you consent to receiving (e.g., bruises, scratches, cuts)?
- Who will be bringing cream, ice packs, etc. to help dress or care for the wounds after the scene?
- Are there particular places on your body where you do not want to be marked? (Some folks allow marks only on parts of their body that will not be seen publicly, such as the butt, breasts, back, or upper thighs).

STI, Disease, and Pregnancy Protection

If any sort of sexual touch or penetration will be included in a kink scene, discussing protection is an important way to keep all participants safe. This includes play that involves blood or the exposure of bodily fluids.

Potential questions could include the following:

- Should sexual contact take place, which forms of protection will we utilize?
- When was the last time you had an STI test? What were the results?

- Are you currently sexually active with other partners? What forms of protection are you using with them?
- Are you comfortable with fluid bonding? If so, does that include ejaculation in the mouth, genitals, or anus?

Past Trauma/Trigger Plans

Sharing personal traumatic experiences is a vulnerable and sometimes frightening experience. If the scene is being planned with a long-term or trusted partner/s, disclosure of past trauma could serve as a way to provide an additional layer of safety or protection to the scene. That said, if the space does not feel safe enough to disclose or share past traumatic experiences, it can still be beneficial to personally note the ways in which past events may influence present or future reactions. There are also many cases where folks are unaware of how their trauma could reactivate during a scene, which can be a terrifying and sometimes confusing experience. A trigger plan is the pre-negotiated action that will be taken if one or more participants in the scene get emotionally activated. It should include what activation historically has looked like; what safe word will be used; what to do immediately following the trigger; and lastly, if play should continue, how folks may re-enter the space.

Potential questions could include the following:

- Have you been activated during a scene before?
- What do you believe triggered the activation?
- Are there positions, movements, language, or settings that may evoke negative past experiences?
- Should a trigger occur, what are the best steps to help move toward a place of regulation?
- Should a trigger occur, how would you like to indicate whether you wish to continue in the scene?

There are many concepts and questions that are not included above that may be essential to negotiate for particular types of scenes. The list should not be the only thing utilized during a negotiation; it is a starting point only and should be based on the preferences, styles, and desires of those participating in the scene. You may have noticed that there is one particularly important concept that was not covered in the list above, and that is aftercare.

Aftercare

Arguably one of the most essential aspects of a kink encounter occurs when the scene comes to an end. Whether sexual or non-sexual, kink scenes tend to elicit a rush of chemicals that can, in some cases, result in an altered physiological state. Moving from the high of the scene back down to a regulated state can be a challenging experience and requires a buffer to lower someone gently back to their psychological and physiological baseline. Aftercare is one of the pillars of kink and, whenever possible, should be integrated into kink scenes, as it is the time when all parties involved have an opportunity to decompress from the scene *in the ways that best suit them*. Indeed, aftercare does not solely belong to the kink community; it is an excellent way to integrate care after all sexual interactions—non-kink included.

Aftercare is person specific; and while there are many ways to integrate it post-play, no one-size-fits-all technique, style, or version will work for everyone. An important note about aftercare is that it is best to discuss and decide on the aftercare plan during the negotiation, *prior* to the scene. Similarly to how people cannot give informed consent to a scene mid-scene, aftercare can be very difficult to plan and integrate while still sitting in the intensity of the scene. Grounded in consent, aftercare exists as a means to nurture all parties after the scene has come to an end.

A variety of emotional, physical, and physiological responses can arise upon completion of a scene, some within minutes and others up to days or weeks later. Kink play often requires a large amount of energy expenditure, so experiencing a wave of exhaustion immediately following a scene is not uncommon or unusual. Often, this physical reaction can be remedied by engaging in aftercare in a way that is replenishing (e.g., food, water, rest); however, a few other more complex reactions all center around the concept of drop:

> The phenomena commonly described as sub drop, Dom drop, or simply drop refer both to the "drop" in energy and mood that many people experience following BDSM/kink headspace or activities and to the psychological after-effects of BDSM/kink experiences . . . drop is a natural physiological consequence following the rush of endorphins and adrenaline that people often experience during BDSM/kink headspaces and activities.
>
> Ansara, 2019

In addition to sub and Dom drop, which typically occur within a relatively close timeframe to the play itself, researchers Sprott and

Randall (2016) have proposed a new type of drop that may help explain what happens when someone experiences a drop days or weeks after a scene:

> We propose that the later kind of x-drop is not a biochemical process as much as it is a process of loss and grief, or a reaction to loss that is part of identity change. Perhaps the later x-drop is a sign of growth, but a growth process that involves negative emotional experiences as part of the change. X-drop becomes the felt aspect of the challenge of incorporating the peak experience into one's life. Or integrating past losses into one's present life. Or it is the felt aspect of identity change. In either case, the experience of drop may be a healthy process and may not be a sign of something going wrong, may not be a sign of pathology or dysfunction.
>
> Sprott & Randall, 2016

It may be confusing to imagine that negative emotions may follow a positive consensual kink scene; however, the idea of having an unexplainable negative response to "vanilla" sex despite the interaction being positive is also present in the literature. Postcoital dysphoria "is a counter-intuitive phenomenon characterized by inexplicable feelings of tearfulness, sadness, or irritability following otherwise satisfactory consensual sexual activity" (Maczkowiack & Schweitzer, 2018). Sometimes, our brains and bodies respond in ways that we do not understand or even like. It is for this reason that aftercare, whether in a kink or non-kink context, is so important.

The following are a variety of ways to engage in aftercare that may be helpful to utilize upon completion of a scene. This list is by no means exhaustive and should be explicitly tailored to whoever is involved in the scene:

- **Massages:** Bonding after a scene is an important aspect of aftercare, bringing the intention back to connection. In addition to increased intimacy, massaging one another can be a great way to lower stress and anxiety.
- **Bathing together:** Another way to increase intimacy, bathing or showering together may be a good way for partners to re-establish connection and clean up!
- **Consuming snacks and rehydrating:** Replenishing with both food and water is a great way to regain energy following a scene, especially one that took a significant amount of physical energy or time. Snacks may also be a reward in certain dynamics to indicate a job well done.

- **Tending to any wounds/injuries acquired during the scene:** A number of kink activities may result in bruises, cuts, and scratches. It is crucial that any wounds/injuries are tended to following a scene.
- **Cuddling:** When engaging in gentle physical touch with a partner, in addition to reduced anxiety and stress, the release of oxytocin—the "feel-good hormone"—elicits feelings of bonding and trust, two incredibly important factors following an intense scene.
- **Words of affirmation:** Re-establishing connection can be vital after a scene that includes any form of humiliation, degradation, or various forms of power play. Coming together after a scene to affirm the experience can be an excellent way not only to increase intimacy but to lessen the temporary shame that sometimes arises when participating in taboo sexual activities.
- **Taking a walk and getting some fresh air:** For some, going for a light walk or stepping outside may be a good way to regulate following a scene. It is important, however, that whoever is going for a walk is psychologically and physically able to do so at the time. For some, this may need to happen after an initial rest period.
- **Using a weighted blanket:** A BDSM scene may result in an elevated heart rate and breathing pattern. Due to the pressure of a weighted blanket, an individual's autonomic nervous system goes into "rest" mode, which can allow for increased feelings of calm and the reduction of anxiety symptoms.
- **Napping:** After a particularly exhausting scene, a nap may be exactly what is needed. The Mayo Clinic notes that napping can offer a number of benefits for healthy adults, including relaxation, improved mood, and reduced fatigue (Mayo Clinic Staff, 2022).

Another facet of aftercare occurs beyond the negotiated aftercare implementation; this part is known as the "debrief." Depending on when all involved parties are ready—emotionally and physically (and this could be the day of the scene or in the following days)—there should be a space to discuss the scene itself. During this conversation, participants can discuss how they felt about the scene, what went well, what they would change in the future, and more. The debrief is a vital part of the kink experience as it affords folks the space to express their feelings about the scene. It can be particularly significant if there were aspects that were not enjoyable. The debrief is the final step in the kink interaction and often will lead back into the negotiation for the next time the parties play. Communication must be woven into all aspects of a scene, and this cycle—negotiation, scene, aftercare, and debriefing—is essential to the kink experience.

ADDITIONAL RESOURCES

Superfreaks: Kink, Pleasure, and the Pursuit of Happiness by Arielle Greenberg

Life, Leather, and the Pursuit of Happiness: Life, History and Culture in the Leather/BDSM/Fetish Community by Steve Lenius

Power Circuits: Polyamory in a Power Dynamic by Raven Kaldera

Playing Well with Others: Your Field Guide to Discovering, Navigating and Exploring the Kink, Leather, and BDSM Communities by Lee Harrington and Mollena Williams

Leather Folk by Mark Thompson (ed.)

8

PROBLEMATIC BEHAVIOR
Elyssa Helfer

THE HISTORY OF CLINICAL BIASES

To truly understand the intense discrimination and stereotyping of kinky folks, it is vital to take a look back in time to uncover not only the inception of kink behavior, but the major turning points that shaped the ways in which kinky desires became seen as non-normative, unnatural, and even pathological. So, let us jump into a quick (or not-so-quick) history lesson. It is challenging to identify the definitive origin point of deliberate BDSM-related sexual activities. There are plenty of points in history when we can see the use of implements similar to those used within a BDSM context today (e.g., whips, floggers); however, questions around intention, pleasure, and notably consent remain.

Perhaps the first graphical depiction of erotic flogging dates back to the 5th century B.C.: what is now called the "Tomb of the Whipping," which was discovered in 1960. However, historian and author of *The History and Arts of the Dominatrix* Anne Nomis suggests that the earliest example of BDSM behavior as part of human history can be found in rites to worship the Mesopotamian Goddess Inanna, around 4000–3100 BC. When examining the infliction of sexual pain, historians have unearthed evidence of diamastigosis—known more commonly as "ritual flagellation"—within Ancient Greek practices dating back to the 9th century B.C. Further, depictions from the years 730–727 BC illustrate the incorporation of whips and floggers in rituals and scenarios of sexual domination. Delving into this historical narrative suggests that the act of whipping might have

DOI: 10.4324/9781003312833-8

had a dual nature, serving both as a sacred and sexual ritual and a punitive measure. However, historical records do not offer conclusive evidence regarding the consensual nature of these acts (Nomis, 2013).

Centuries later, traces of what we would consider modern-day kink persisted in historical settings and literature—notably exemplified in the *Kama Sutra*. As the oldest surviving Hindu text on eroticism and sexuality (Doniger, 2003), the *Kama Sutra* explored the synthesis of pain and pleasure. Moreover, it underscored the ethical principle that activities such as impact play and other BDSM interactions should only involve individuals who understand the dynamics involved and, more crucially, willingly consent to such experiences (Vatsyayana, 1883). What we would now consider kinky activities seemed to pop up around the world for thousands of years. However, it is simply not possible to conflate historical kinky behavior with what we see today as kink, as the aspect of consent may not have been present. The kink that we understand today came about much more recently and was heavily influenced by the history of libertinism.

As philosophical libertinism gained momentum in 17th-century France, a culture of pushing against the status quo began to emerge, particularly in the realm of sexual expression and the pursuit of pleasure. Libertines—defined today as people, particularly men, "who [behave] without moral principles or a sense of responsibility, especially in sexual matters" (Oxford Dictionary)—questioned the attitudes, and further the laws, around sex and sexual morality. The Enlightenment (1685–1815) was a period in which an emphasis on critical thinking, libertarianism, and the pursuit of science began shifting sociocultural perspectives and challenging the motivation for the inheritance of moral law from scripture. However, the movement away from sexual morality being a philosophical problem reframed non-normative sex as a medical problem instead, introducing barbaric forms of medical intervention both in and out of asylums (Hart & Wellings, 2002).

Non-normative sexual behavior and desires thus shifted from a moral issue to a medical issue and ultimately moved into the realm of psychiatry, thus introducing the concept of clinical pathologization. The current pathologization of non-normative sexual behaviors was undoubtedly influenced by the Victorian Era's rigid definition of "normal" sex (heterosexual, romantic, private, married, suburban, and monogamous); and was further amplified by the noteworthy beliefs of Richard von Krafft Ebing (1840–1902)—also known as the Father of Modern Sexology—and Albert Moll (1862–1939). The late 1800s ushered in a time when differentiating normative and non-normative sexual interests became central areas of focus:

> From around 1870, psychiatrists shifted the focus from immoral acts, a temporary deviation of the norm, to an innate morbid condition. In the late nineteenth century, several psychiatrists, collecting and publishing more and more case histories, classified and explained the wide range of deviant sexual behaviours they traced . . . Their main thrust was that in many cases, irregular sexual behavior should not be regarded as sin and crime but as symptoms of pathology . . . The emergence of medical sexology meant that perversions could be diagnosed and discussed.
>
> Oosterhuis, 2012

While several early sexologists had an influence on what has become modern-day clinical pathologization, von Krafft-Ebing's 1886 work, *Psychopatia Sexualis*, marked a critical turning point in the development of clinical biases surrounding kink. Influenced by Leopold von Sacher-Masoch's works entitled *Venus in Furs* and the Marquis de Sade's *Justine, Juliette, and 120 Days of Sodom*, von Krafft-Ebing coined the terms "sadism" and "masochism," officially creating the first "diagnosable" BDSM-related activities. von Krafft-Ebing, however, was not simply known for the introduction of new sex-related terminology; his writing also paved the way for a new type of pathologization—one that conflated "unapproved sexual activities" with psychiatric complications (Shorter, 2014). Prior to his work, sexual practices that fell outside the conventional norm were considered expressions of "insanity"; however, due to his medicalization of sexual deviance, psychiatry became a necessity for those who held or acted upon these deviant behaviors or desires. Interestingly, von Krafft-Ebing's belief that these "perversions" were "proof of genetic weakness" was heavily influenced by both his inability to acknowledge the sexual agency of women and his concern that the "degenerates" who possessed these traits could cause problems that would interfere with evolutionary fitness, particularly in the realm of procreation (Shorter, 2014).

It is clear that by this point in history, the idea that it could be healthy for women to desire sex for the sake of pleasure or that sexual sadism or masochism could be healthy forms of expression was entirely unfathomable. It did not help that Freud's 1905 work, *Three Essays on the Theory of Sexuality*, reinforced the idea that sadomasochism (a term which he coined by combining "sadism" and "masochism") required psychiatric treatment. Freud continued to push the idea that non–normative expressions of sexuality were indeed a perversion. The narratives that fueled the pathologization of sexual behavior continued throughout the early 1900s and undoubtedly influenced what would ultimately become the formal classification of "sexual deviation," a diagnosis in the *DSM-I* within the "socio-pathic personality disturbance" category of personality disorders. (The *DSM* and its profound influence on clinical and cultural biases will be discussed in depth later in this chapter.)

Fortunately, thanks to the many sexual revolutionaries who kick-started the American Sexual Revolution in the 1960s, the concep-tualizations around kink behavior did begin to shift slowly. As more people—including sex researchers—began to question how much the concept of morality influenced views on sex and sexuality, a new world of exploration opened up. Questions surrounding the con-cept of "healthy" kink shifted away from being both a psychiatric and philosophical issue to determining if it was a psychological issue. Spoiler alert: decades of kink research have indicated time and time again that it is not.

WHAT COUNTS AS NORMAL?

As more and more kink-related concepts have been presented throughout this book, you may have noticed yourself wondering: is any of this normal? For centuries, there have been shifting views of what constitutes normal sexual behavior and, pretty consist-ently, kink has fallen outside of those lines. Today, there are plenty of resources presenting statistics on sexual behavior and interests

Scan to view the Kinsey Institute's Sex FAQs & Information.

Figure 8.1   Sex FAQs & Information from the Kinsey Institute (QR code)

(the Kinsey Institute's Sex FAQS is a great example). Even within the pages of this book, we have given percentages and research participant data suggesting what the sexual landscape currently looks like concerning BDSM. That said, one of the more complex issues surrounding the understanding of sexual behavior is that the idea of "normal" does not hold as much weight as it once did. What is considered normal will vary between different cultures, age groups, relationship structures, and more. When it comes to BDSM, given the various research studies suggesting that "fantasies [about BDSM are] found to be common (40–70%)" (Brown et al., 2020), some could argue that kink desires are generally "normal" and that not having any kink desires is "abnormal." That said, claiming that something is "normal" or "not normal" based solely on numbers gathered at a specific time, from specific participants in specific places, while scientifically sound, completely erases the nuance of individual experience. It does not consider the fluidity of the subjectivity of "normalcy," which shifts depending on context, settings, moods, relationship structures, etc.

One helpful example of the fluidity of "normal" is the use of porn (we will thoroughly discuss porn use later in this chapter). Utilizing porn may be completely acceptable and even encouraged in one relationship and completely off the table in another. If over half of the population have watched porn at some point in their lives (Cox et al., 2022), we may be able to argue that watching porn is normal—right? Well, not exactly. If porn is off the table and one partner nonetheless watches porn, while they may be participating in something that is arguably considered "normal," they are also breaking a relationship agreement, which induces feelings of betrayal, hurt, and resentment. So, while watching porn can be considered a generally normal experience, that is not particularly relevant to the person who has just been betrayed by their partner. In this relationship, watching porn is not normal. In fact, what this couple would consider normal is refraining from watching porn. Thus, there is a difference between what is "normal" in the grander scheme of someone's life versus what is "normal" within a particular relationship and even what is "normal" clinically. Further, we must be very clear that when it comes to consensual interactions between adults, "normal" will naturally differ from person to person; and fundamentally, when it comes to sexual desire and behavior, the question that should be considered is not "What is normal?" but rather "What is problematic?"

The first primary differentiating factor when considering what is problematic sexual behavior is a lack of consent. If anyone is engaging in non-consensual behavior, we can safely say that we have moved into problematic territory. This especially applies when someone of adult age is sexually engaging with a minor. While state-to-state laws differ regarding the age of consent, non-consent is always a problem when it comes to minors; and even with consent gained by participating parties, there remains an abundance of reasons why that type of engagement can be problematic. The next factor to consider is the extent to which a desire or behavior is causing personal distress—in particular, if the desire or behavior is impacting someone's ability to function in different aspects of their life. Is their desire resulting in such severe rumination that they are unable to complete tasks at work? Does their behavior seem out of control to the point that they are risking personal safety to engage in that behavior? These are the types of questions we may ask ourselves when trying to understand if what we desire is indeed problematic.

We also want to consider that there is a difference between wanting or desiring something and actually engaging in it. In my clinical practice, I often help clients work through shame regarding their desires, which is particularly relevant when those desires fall into problematic or criminal categories. One analogy that I frequently bring into the therapeutic space is intended to illustrate that our desires do not identify us: if someone is standing at the counter at a bank and is tempted to steal the cash as they watch the bank teller count out a stack of $100 bills, it does not mean that they are a bank robber. The criminal desire they hold becomes a crime only when they act out the desire. Thus, wanting to rob a bank, thinking of robbing a bank, or even wishing they could rob a bank does not mean they are doomed to end up a bank robber; it means that work must be done to ensure they do not act on that desire. While this example involves a desire that falls under the criminal category—one where the act could be punishable by law—there are other types of desires that folks struggle with because they feel, with certainty, that they are just "wrong."

For many, the shame surrounding a particular desire may not necessarily be because engaging in that behavior would be criminal. In fact, for many, engaging in their desire with another consenting adult could be incredibly fulfilling and enjoyable. The problem here lies in the perceived judgment stemming from social and cultural stigma. Given the significant history of pathologizing sexual desire and behaviors, it is unsurprising that stigma-influenced shame is a pressing concern for many kinky people—particularly if they have not been exposed to other kinky folks or have grown up in a sexually repressive environment. Without a community to normalize behavior or a system in place to allow access to kink education, someone can grow up believing that they are alone in their desires due to the missed opportunity of seeking community. As we continue to dive deeper into understanding problematic sexual behavior, we must keep in mind the intense influence that societal stigma and shame have on individuals' beliefs about themselves.

MASTURBATION

> Modern masturbation is profane. It is not just something that putatively makes those who do it tired, crippled, mad, or blind but an act with serious ethical implications. It is that part of human sexual life where potentially unlimited pleasure meets social restraint, where habit and the promise of just-one-more-time struggle with the dictates of conscience and good sense; where fantasy silences, if only for a moment, the reality principle; and where the autonomous self escapes from the erotically barren here and now into a luxuriant world of its own creation. It hovers between abjection and fulfillment.
>
> —Laqueur, 2003

As Laqueur notes in his book *Solitary Sex: A Cultural History of Masturbation*, the conversation around engagement in masturbation is a complicated one, filled with competing beliefs, strong opinions, and the perpetuation of myths. Fundamentally, there is no universal definition of "masturbation," although most can agree that masturbation involves stimulating one's genitals for sexual pleasure. That said, what is more important to take into consideration is not a general definition of "masturbation" but rather how each individual relates to or engages in the practice. Researchers Kirschbaum and Peterson (2017) emphasize several important factors to take into account when considering an individual's personal definition of and relationship with masturbation. These include personal variables—such as personal history and experiences with masturbation, demographics, individual attitudes, and beliefs—and situational factors (Kirschbaum & Peterson, 2017). This is particularly vital when trying to determine whether masturbation is a problem.

Similar to the ways in which sadism and masochism were medicalized as psychiatric issues in the late 1800s, engaging in masturbation was also believed to result in insanity and a plethora of other severe health conditions (Laqueur, 2003). Myths surrounding masturbation's impact on both physical and mental health have continued to penetrate the sociocultural landscape despite evidence to suggest a variety of positive mental and physical health outcomes for those who engage in masturbation (Coleman, 2002; Shulman & Horne, 2003).

> Masturbation continued to be a morally fraught, much-thought-about arena of human sexuality—indeed a critical component of what came to be understood as "sexuality"—long after it stopped being regarded as a cause of real physical harm. It remains so today, even though its most virulent opponents no longer claim that it causes blindness, madness, or other bodily ills. Moral passion and medical danger grew up together, the latter as an expression of the former. But when the threat of physical harm ceased to be persuasive, the anxiety about solitary sex—first voiced in 1712—did not go away. To the contrary.
>
> Laqueur, 2003

When determining whether any sexual behavior or interest is problematic, one cannot overlook the impact of historical views on the current culture and how those may have shaped overarching views about what some may consider "taboo" topics. Understanding how the roles of shame, fear, and judgment may be a deterrent to self-pleasure gives us insight into the individual experiences and perspectives of problematic masturbation. While there are a number of reasons why someone might engage in masturbation (which we will cover below), noting the reasons why someone may *not* engage shines a light on the impacts of how external forces can guide and shape belief systems. Aside from a lack of privacy (this is a common one!), many individuals also refrain due to cultural shame, medical misinformation, religious shame or prohibition, social stigma, as well as disapproval from partners (Carvalheira & Leal, 2013; Cito et al., 2021; Kaestle & Allen, 2011; Lester et al., 2016; Walsh, 2000; Laqueur, 2003).

It is nearly impossible to research masturbation without considering the profound impact that religious affiliation has had on beliefs that masturbation is a sin. Throughout history, both religious groups and cultural communities have prohibited masturbation due to the lack of possibility of procreation and, further, its primary focus on pleasure (Buaban, 2021; Bullough, 2003; Huang, 2023). Given these reasons, it comes as no surprise that significant internal conflict can arise should someone be interested in masturbation when it is clouded by accusations of sin. Whether it is prohibited by someone's religious beliefs or by their romantic partner, the weight of the shame for having the desire to masturbate can undoubtedly contribute to making some people feel as though something is wrong with them or that their desires are problematic.

When trying to determine and assess whether masturbation might be problematic, the following questions can be considered.

Is Masturbation Itself the Problem?

This question, as a whole, is not possible to answer due to the nuance that must be considered when evaluating one's masturbation habits. For the most part, problems with masturbation are subjective and can vary from person to person; however, they are typically due to behavior which is *related* to masturbation, not the masturbation itself (although this is not always the case—see further below). While there are certainly many instances of shame and guilt being associated with masturbation, there are also various positive effects and experiences related to masturbation. Throughout the years, both within academic settings and in the popular media, abundant reasons for participating in masturbation have been presented. Let's start with why someone might masturbate in the first place. Researchers have found that people may masturbate to:

- release sexual tension;
- feel sexual pleasure;
- experience an orgasm;
- learn more about their own body;
- help fall asleep;
- work on self-love;
- make up for having less partnered sex than they prefer;
- ease pain;
- reduce stress;
- boost mood; and
- enhance their sex life (Bowman, 2014, Cleveland Clinic, 2022; Herbenick et al 2023; Fahs & Frank, 2014; Regnerus et al, 2017, Rowland et al., 2020,)

Is Masturbation a Physical Problem?

Masturbation involves interaction with extremely sensitive parts of the human body and not being mindful of the ways in which those parts are engaged with can result in physical harm or injury. For example, excessive rubbing or utilizing hands or toys without adequate lubrication can result in skin irritation, rashes, broken skin, and genital discomfort or swelling. Utilizing lubrication, ensuring that hands and toys are clean before insertion, and stopping or adjusting when skin irritation begins are a few ways to help prevent physical injury. Suppose someone continues to engage in masturbation despite experiencing physical pain or injury. In that case, it may be indicative of problematic behavior related to masturbation, as they are actively engaging in self-harm. At that point, they may want to consider consulting with a professional.

So, to return to our original question: is masturbation a physical problem? It certainly can be. Does this mean that masturbation is a problem? Not necessarily. It means that education, intention, and bodily awareness are factors to keep in mind if someone chooses to engage in masturbation. Being mindful of the ways that masturbation can result in physical harm and minimizing those risks can be an excellent way to stay outside of "problematic" territory.

Is Masturbation a Relational Problem?

We cannot simply categorize engagement in occasional or regular masturbation while in a committed romantic relationship as a problem. There are plenty of couples, triads, and other relationship configurations in which masturbation is welcomed, encouraged, or simply neutral. When masturbation begins to become a problem, it typically has to do with the overall relational dynamics. Within the context of a romantic relationship—whether with one or more partners—agreements are made with the expectation that all parties involved will adhere to the agreed-upon boundaries. Masturbation becomes a relational problem if all parties agree to abstain from masturbating and someone violates that boundary.

Another problem that can arise is when one partner prefers masturbation to engaging sexually or intimately with their partner. Again, this does not necessarily mean that there is a problem with masturbation (although it can be; we will get to that soon). This can often be indicative of a greater relational issue; or—and this may not be easy to digest—masturbation may be that person's preferred mode of sex (solo sex) and the relational "issue" is one of sexual incompatibility. In these cases, while masturbation may be the behavioral action taken, the underlying issues can be far more complex. Trust is violated when a relationship agreement is broken and the reasons for that violation are essential to explore. When one partner prefers masturbation to sex with their partner, it may be an issue of incompatibility, sexual disconnection, or more.

Let us look deeper into the concept of relationship agreements. Imagine that Jennifer and Melissa are in a long-term monogamous relationship. They have regular sex and are overall very happy in their relationship. Due to [fill in the blank] reason, Melissa believes that masturbation is akin to cheating, and after expressing this to Jennifer, *both* partners have agreed that they will not engage in masturbation. If Jennifer masturbates, she is violating the relationship agreement, breaking Melissa's trust and crossing a well-established boundary. Whether or not Jennifer feels that masturbation is a problem itself, the relationship has now experienced a rupture that will need to be repaired. In a case like this, it may be easy to ascribe the problem to masturbation. However, this is fundamentally a matter of violated boundaries and could have happened due to a number of different behaviors.

Is Masturbation a Psychological Problem?

There is no evidence to suggest that masturbation causes mental health disorders. That said, could a depression diagnosis shift the way someone engages with their body? Absolutely. Could anxiety result in a struggle to achieve orgasm? Totally. Could depression symptoms arise if someone has moral objections to masturbation yet desires or engages with it? Yes. While there may be correlations between masturbation and mental health diagnoses, this does not indicate causation. Remember, correlation does not imply causation (as every high-school science teacher has said).

> The psychological interpretation of people's masturbation behavior is essential. Some people masturbate often but do not regard this as problematic. On the other hand, some do not necessarily have a high masturbation frequency, but they may consider themselves masturbating too much and thus fall in the problematic masturbation category.
>
> Huang et al., 2023

While the questions above may feel somewhat complicated, the overall point is that masturbation itself is typically not a problem. The problems begin to arise when:

- the desire to masturbate is feeling out of control or the behavior is compulsive;
- masturbation is causing psychological distress, whether due to personal, moral, social, or cultural conflict;
- masturbation is getting in the way of daily functioning (e.g., missing work, staying up all night);
- masturbation within a relational context is violating a relationship agreement;
- excessive or intense masturbation is causing physical injury or discomfort; or
- any combination of the above.

Overall, there are many ways in which masturbation can be integrated into someone's life in a healthy, fulfilling, and pleasurable way. As a way to engage in sexual pleasure without the risk of STIs or unwanted pregnancy, it is undeniably one of the safest forms of sexual engagement. Guilt and shame may be attributed to masturbation; however, when this happens, we must look at the bigger picture to find the source.

PORNOGRAPHY

In 2022, Alan McKee, Katerina Litsou, Paul Byron, and Roger Ingham released an analysis of the insights gained after half a century of cross-disciplinary research into pornography. Their findings were scathing: they identified inconsistencies in defining "pornography"; ongoing biases in research; reporting of correlations unsupported by their findings; the framing of inquiries from a position that normalized "Charmed Circle" standards; and a failure to interpret data in ways that acknowledged the possibility of healthy alternative sexualities and relationships (McKee et al., 2010). One of their most important observations, for our purposes, was the way in which consensual BDSM was consistently framed as problematic behavior within the studies they reviewed: "Discussion of consent often falls within research about pornography's relationship with sexual violence. And much of this research does not distinguish between non-consensual violence, and consensual practices of BDSM, kink, spanking, role playing, and rough sex" (ibid).

This operational deficit can become a self-fulfilling cycle in clinical application; when one defines depictions of BDSM as intrinsically violent, one is more likely to perceive a connection between pornography viewing and "violent" behavior in the viewer. This can result in microaggressions and stigma toward kinky clients who may feel seen and validated by depictions of their own relational and erotic practices within the context of erotic media, as well as in the misdiagnosis of otherwise healthy behaviors as problematic, addictive, or maladaptive. McKee et al. reemphasized the lack of empirical foundation that we have for these fears, writing that:

> it remains the case that no simple conclusions can be drawn about associations between consuming (various kinds of) pornography and (various kinds of) (non-)consensual sexual behaviors. Despite this fact, many recent articles display an unwarranted confidence that the state of knowledge in regard to pornography consumption and consent is more settled than is in fact the case.
>
> McKee, Litsou, Byron, & Ingham, 2022

Setting aside the idea of pornography being somehow linked to one's kink identity or BDSM expression, we must still acknowledge that many people express concern about the viewing of erotic content at all—regardless of whether it is thematically kinky. The reality is that humans have been creating and consuming erotic content since we first picked up a charred twig to sketch on the walls of a cave and will likely continue to do so with whatever form of technology enters our lives for the foreseeable future. Marty Klein, in his book *His Porn, Her Pain,* discusses asking the following questions when working to determine if pornography use has become problematic (Klein, 2016):

- **Is the problem porn or is it the internet?** How connected are you to your devices? Do you feel uncomfortable disconnecting from the online world? Do you feel a sense of urgency when you see a push notification on your phone? Are these answers true regardless of whether you have been watching online porn?
- **Is the problem porn or is it masturbation?** What messages did you receive about self-pleasure growing up? Do you believe that masturbation can be a healthy part of one's private (or relational) life? Do you feel guilt or shame about your masturbation?

Do you prefer masturbation to sex with your partner(s)? Are these answers true regardless of whether you have been viewing porn?

- **Is the problem porn or is the sexual dynamics in your relationship(s)?** Do you have satisfying sex with your partner(s)? Do you feel comfortable and confident in your sexual skills? Do you feel desire for, and desired by, your partner(s)? Do you have the opportunity to explore your sexual fantasies within your relationship? Are these answers the same regardless of whether you have been watching porn?
- **Is the problem porn or is porn being used to mediate anxiety, depression, loneliness, or anger?** Do you find yourself watching more content when you are bored? Do you seek out media that shows you a relationship style, sexual practice, or power dynamic that you want for yourself? Do you talk about your feelings and desires with your partner(s)? Do you have friends in your life who share your relationship style or power dynamic preferences? Are these answers true regardless of whether you have been watching porn?

There is no empirical evidence that pornography use itself is problematic. There is even less data linking pornography to problematic sexual behaviors or sexual violence—as we have seen, where this seems to be the case, it is more often an instance of anti-kink stigma informing the data analysis. Likewise, there is no evidence that erotic media comprises an addictive substance that inevitably leads people toward more unethical/problematic content:

> Scientists Gaddam and Ogas examined the Google searches of thousands of people and found that overwhelmingly, they have fixed, unchanging sexual interests and search for porn of the same type, over and over again. Sex and porn do not create a slippery slope—which leads people to seek out more and more perverse porn as they get bored with more mundane images. Instead, people, especially men, get pretty stuck on a few, restricted types of images, scenes, and fantasies.
>
> Ley, 2016

Ultimately, we can say the following about pornography in the context of our understanding of problematic behaviors:

- The research that has been conducted over the last 50 years has not identified a definitive causal link between the use of erotic media (of all kinds) and problematic sexual or relational behaviors.

- "Self-reported addiction to pornography is probably deeply intertwined with religious and moral beliefs for some people . . . When people morally disapprove of pornography but still use it anyway, they are more likely to report that pornography is interfering with their lives" (Grubbs, 2020). This is a reaction known as "moral incongruence."
- Many of the studies that claim to have found such links are grounded in a fundamental lack of kink competency and anti-BDSM stigma that inform and influence the conclusions that they reach.

ETHICAL NON-MONOGAMY

In Western culture, an idealized view of monogamy prevails, resulting in significant stigmatization and discrimination toward folks whose relational styles do not conform to the notion that both sexual and romantic connections must exist exclusively with one partner (Moors et al., 2021). Ethical non-monogamy—sometimes known as "consensual non-monogamy" or simply as an "open relationship"— is an umbrella of relational styles that can include being in a romantic and sometimes sexual relationship with more than one person. While the terms "ethical" and "consensual" are currently being reevaluated within non-monogamous communities, as non-monogamy without consent is what many consider cheating, they remain widely utilized by those within and outside of the community. Being in a non-monogamous relationship means that all parties are abreast of the relational engagement of all partners. Similar to the kink community, consent, negotiation, and communication are all crucial to engaging in this dynamic in a healthy way. Fundamentally, "non-monogamy" is an umbrella term encompassing a plethora of relational constellations.

There are various ways to engage in non-monogamy, mainly as these relationship structures are often built on the needs and desires of the participants. While there certainly are ways that each type is defined, like kink, there is no one-size-fits-all way to participate in non-monogamy—with the exception of ensuring informed consent. Polyamory expert Dr. Elisabeth Sheff described a few of the more common relationship structures as follows (Sheff, 2014):

- **Swinging:** "Swinging involves committed couples consensually exchanging partners specifically for sexual purposes. It is tremendously diverse, ranging from brief interactions between or among strangers at sex parties or clubs, to groups of friends who know each other and have socialized for many years."

- **Polyamory:** Polyamory is "a relationship style that allows people to openly conduct multiple sexual and/or romantic relationships simultaneously, ideally with the knowledge and consent of all involved in or affected by the relationships."
- **Monogamish:** "Popularized within the last few years by Dan Savage, monogamish relationships are those in which a couple is primarily monogamous but allows varying degrees of sexual contact with others. As with other non-monogamous relationships, rules structuring these external sexual contacts vary by couple."
- **Relationship anarchy:** "Due to the anarchist nature of this relationship philosophy, it is difficult to pin down an exact definition of relationship anarchy (RA), but two themes appear regularly in the writings of people who discuss it. First, relational anarchists are often highly critical of conventional cultural standards that prioritize romantic and sex-based relationships over non-sexual or non-romantic relationships. Instead, RA seeks to eliminate specific distinctions between or hierarchical valuations of friendships versus love-based relationships, so that love-based relationships are no more valuable than platonic friendships. Second, another important theme within RA is the resistance to placing demands or expectations on the people involved in a relationship. Whereas swingers and polyamorists often create specific rules and guidelines to structure their relationships, RA rejects such rules as inevitably leading to a hierarchical valuation of some partners over others. In RA, no one should have to give anything up or compromise in order to sustain a relationship; rather, it is better to amicably separate than to sustain an unhappy and unfulfilling relationship."

Everywhere you turn, loud voices are screaming that non-monogamy as a whole is a problem. As deeply embedded in mononormative culture as we are, there has been a pervasive shaming of non-monogamous folks, resulting in not only emotional distress but a variety of negative consequences (remember, like kink, non-monogamy as an identity is not a protected class, which means non-monogamous folks are often targets of discrimination). When we start to consider if non-monogamy in itself is a problem, we may begin to see a pattern here. It is not often the non-monogamy itself that can be problematic; it is how people engage with it.

So when, if at all, does non-monogamy become problematic?

Have you ever heard a person say that they are non-monogamous, but they have not disclosed it to the person they are dating and have other partners on the side? I certainly have; and this is the type of behavior that paints a negative picture of what non-monogamy actually is. This type of relationship is not grounded in consent, puts folks at risk (especially if sexually active), and is essentially based on false information. In a case like this, non-monogamy is being weaponized as a means to engage in multiple non-consensual partnerships, and the problem here is far from the structure of the relationship. Any version of non-monogamy where folks are not disclosing other partnerships (unless this is pre-negotiated) is problematic; however, it is the communication—or lack thereof—that is truly the problem. In addition, there are folks who attempt to engage in non-monogamous relationships and find that while they believe in the relationship style, they are unable to feel entirely safe within their relationships. Non-monogamy is not for everyone, and trying to fit oneself into a structure that does not authentically resonate can result in significant emotional distress. Again, this issue is not related to non-monogamy itself; it is connected to engaging in a behavior that is fundamentally uncomfortable and misaligned. As you can see, lack of consent and personal distress are two clear indicators of problematic behavior (we will get into the third indicator later in this chapter), and this does apply to relational structures. Non-monogamy can be an excellent, fulfilling way to connect and relate to others; and it can and often does pair beautifully with kink dynamics.

PARAPHILIAS AND THE *DSM*

The last few years have ushered in a time when diagnoses are not only made within a clinical setting but thrown around within the context of popular media. As trends shift, so does the diagnosis buzzword of the year. While it can certainly feel validating to project or assume someone's potential diagnosis, when it comes to paraphilias in particular, a diagnosis can not only be socially harmful but result in significant emotional, clinical, or even legal consequences. In the matter of kink engagement, decades of research continue to support the theory that there is no single causal factor influencing an interest in BDSM (Brown et al., 2020); nor is there evidence to suggest that these interests are inherently a result of traumatic experiences (Hillier, 2018; Ritchers et al., 2008). In fact, various positive outcomes have been noted in research across the last few decades.

Despite significant stigma and beliefs that BDSM practice is associated with psychopathology, research suggests that practitioners of BDSM do not exhibit higher levels of psychopathology than nonpractitioners, and may actually exhibit higher levels of subjective well-being and lower levels of psychological distress than individuals from the general population. Research also suggests that individuals who engage in BDSM activities may demonstrate higher levels of sexual satisfaction and that BDSM play may serve to enhance relationships.

Jansen et al., 2021

Even with growing evidence to suggest otherwise, the lingering pathologization and stigmatization of kinksters remain strong—in large part due to the unfortunate reality that non-normative sexual behaviors and interests are not only seen as unusual but formally categorized as disordered. While pathologizing non-normative sexual interests existed far prior to the *DSM*'s debut, this marked the beginning of the standardization of sexual behavior in the form of formal diagnoses. According to the American Psychological Association:

The Diagnostic and Statistical Manual of Mental Disorders (DSM) is the handbook used by health care professionals in the United States and much of the world as the authoritative guide to the diagnosis of mental disorders. DSM contains descriptions, symptoms and other criteria for diagnosing mental disorders. It provides a common language for clinicians to communicate about their patients and establishes consistent and reliable diagnoses that can be used in research on mental disorders. It also provides a common language for researchers to study the criteria for potential future revisions and to aid in the development of medications and other interventions.

American Psychological Association

The *DSM* was first published in 1952, following the push for standardizing "disordered" behaviors when US psychiatry gained recognition as a global leader after World War II. From that point and up until the current *DSM-5*, there have been a variety of shifts in how non-normative sexual behaviors have been diagnosed, influenced heavily by the sociocultural landscape at the time of each subsequent release. The *DSM-III*, released in 1980, introduced paraphilias as a subset of the psychosexual disorders. Originally attributed to Friedrich Salomon Krauss (1859–1938), who defined "paraphilias" as "inverted erotic interests," the term was introduced to the English language by sexologist William F. Robinson (1913) and was described by Karpman (1951) as a more objected, scientifically correct term than the word "perversion" (Beech et al., 2016). A "paraphilia" is currently defined as "an intense and persistent sexual interest other than sexual interest in genital stimulation or preparatory fondling with phenotypically normal, physically mature, consenting humans" (Bhatia & Parekh, 2023). To put it simply, it is a sexual interest that falls outside of the "conventional norm." For many years, the desire for non-normative sexual engagement (e.g., sexual masochism or sadism) could result in a paraphilia diagnosis. On the surface, receiving a diagnosis regarding a sexual interest may not seem to hold much weight; however, that is far from the case. From loss of work to loss of child custody, a paraphilia diagnosis has the potential for severe personal and social consequences.

Thanks in large part to the unrelenting efforts of kink advocates and supporters—most notably the NCSF—there was a fight to depathologize consensual sexual behavior by shifting the diagnostic criteria from "paraphilia" to "paraphilic disorder" in the *DSM-5* (Wright, 2010). While these terms appear similar, the differentiation between the two is vital in understanding how this shift became such a powerful step forward for the kink community. Whereas "paraphilia" refers to the interest itself, "paraphilic disorders" are defined as:

> recurrent, intense sexually arousing fantasies, sexual urges, or behaviors that cause distress or impairment to the individual whose satisfaction has entailed personal harm or risk of harm to others, generally involving: non-human objects, the suffering or humiliation of oneself or one's partner, children, or non-consenting persons.
>
> American Psychological Association, 2013

While it may seem subtle, this shift in language has had a profound impact on the kink community because "the distinction between paraphilias and disorders reflects the idea that many people may practice atypical sexual behaviors without meriting a diagnosis of mental illness" (Moran, 2013). However, while this has certainly moved the needle in the pursuit of sexual freedom, there remains a long way to go:

> Although the more formal separation of a paraphilia from a paraphilic disorder may have some immediate effect on the discrimination that individuals with a paraphilia face in civil courts (see Wright, 2010), it surely will not address all the problems these diagnoses have engendered . . . Having a paraphilia has been used to support the discrimination (social, occupational, and legal) against those individuals so designated, despite the lack of data to support their inclusion as a mental disorder.
>
> Moser, 2016

In addition to this shift in the name of and criteria for this diagnosis, the *DSM-5* is notably the first version of the manual in which a distinction is made between paraphilias that are anomalous target preferences and those that are anomalous sexual preferences. Anomalous sexual preferences are further divided into courtship disorders and algolagnic disorders:

> Courtship disorders refer to a construct in sexology in which various anomalous erotic preferences are seen as potentially indicating an underlying disorder (Freund, 1990); Algolagnic Disorders involve the particular paraphilias where sexual arousal is dependent on pain and suffering.
>
> Beech et al., 2016

Let's break this down further.

Figure 8.2 describes one way in which this classification of disorders can be categorized. Another is by looking at which expressions involve criminal behaviors and which do not. For example, paraphilias such as sexual masochism, sexual sadism, fetishism, and transvestism all fall under the category of paraphilias that do not involve criminal behaviors (of course, with the exception of non-consent). On the other hand, voyeurism, frotteurism, exhibitionism, and pedophilia are all paraphilias that are constituted by criminal behavior. We will explore each of these diagnoses in-depth later in the chapter.

While practicing kink in a consensual, ethical, and mindful way can be a healthy form of relational and sexual expression, a number of sexual and relational behaviors are considered problematic and fall

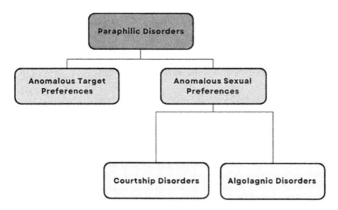

Figure 8.2   Paraphilic Disorders

outside of the realm of kink. One of the primary sources of stigmatization toward the kink community is when those behaviors are still considered kink and the criminal behaviors start to become associated with kinksters as a community. Due to this conflation, many kink academics and experts advocate for the removal of kink desires and behaviors from the *DSM* altogether.

> The history of psychiatry's encounter with sexual diagnoses calls into question the role of psychiatrists as society's moral gatekeepers, one for which the study of histiocytes in medical school poorly qualifies them. The history of the DSM's otherworldly, judgmental, and completely unscientific approach to sex would be risible if the consequences in the real world of making behavior into medical diagnoses were not so serious: for example, partners in divorce cases risk losing access to their children on the grounds that their sexual behavior qualifies them as "perverts" (First, 2014). It's time for psychiatry to bow out of the bedroom.
>
> Shorter, 2014

The Paraphilic Disorders

The following information is derived from a National Library of Medicines article entitled "Paraphilias: Definition, diagnosis and treatment." To differentiate between atypical sexual interest and a mental disorder, the *DSM-5* requires that for diagnosis, people with such interests exhibit the following:

- personal distress about their interest, not merely distress resulting from society's disapproval; or
- a sexual desire or behavior that involves another person's psychological distress, injury, or death, or a desire for sexual behaviors involving unwilling persons or persons unable to give legal consent (McManus et al., 2013).

Anonymous Sexual Preferences: Algolagnic Disorders

- **Sexual masochism disorder:** Sexual masochism disorder manifests as persistent sexual arousal derived from being made to suffer from experiencing physical violence or humiliation. It may include the desire to be beaten, bound, verbally abused, or asphyxiated. Differentiating sexual masochism disorder from a "disorder" and an interest lies in the experience of impairment or distress for the individual. Should negative feelings, shame, and guilt not accompany these desires, the criteria for a diagnosis are not met.

- **Sexual sadism disorder:** Sexual sadism disorder is characterized by sexual arousal resulting from the physical or psychological suffering of another person. This particular disorder manifests as heightened sexual arousal when fantasizing about or observing someone else experiencing physical or psychological pain. While the diagnosis of sexual sadism disorder is appropriate when these urges are acted upon with a non-consenting person, it may also be appropriate to diagnose when these urges are acted upon with a consenting individual if these recurrent desires and behaviors are causing significant distress or impairment in functioning.

Anomalous Target Preferences

- **Fetishistic disorder:** Fetishistic disorder is diagnosed when individuals experience sexual arousal from objects or specific body parts that are not commonly considered erotic, accompanied by acting on particular urges, as well as experiencing distress or an impairment in functioning. According to Beech and Harkins (2012), the most common fetishistic targets are female underwear, feet, and shoes.
- **Transvestic disorder:** Transvestic disorder manifests as sexual arousal as a result of cross-dressing of the opposite gender while experiencing distress about the arousal. An important distinction is that cross-dressing in this particular case is not influenced by gender dysphoria as individuals identify with their gender assigned at birth. Distress or impairment in functioning must accompany the sexual fantasies, urges, and behaviors that are associated with cross-dressing in order for a diagnosis to be appropriate.
- **Pedophilic disorder:** Pedophilic disorder is characterized by an adult—defined as 16 years or older and at least five years older than the child—having intense and recurrent sexual urges, fantasies, or behaviors with prepubescent children (13 years or younger). While the diagnosis is appropriate for individuals who have acted upon their sexual desires—which is a criminal offense—it may also be appropriate for those who are experiencing significant distress due to their desires but have never acted upon them.

Anomalous Sexual Preferences: Courtship Disorders

- **Voyeuristic disorder:** Voyeuristic disorder is characterized by sexual arousal and gratification resulting from observing others engaging in private intimate activities, such as performing sexual acts, being naked, or getting undressed. There are instances where the target is aware of and consents to the voyeur's presence; however, in many cases, the voyeur intentionally engages in such behavior without seeking the target's consent. Differentiating consensual voyeurism as a sexual interest and disorder lies in whether the behaviors or urges are causing an impairment to functioning or significant distress.
- **Exhibitionistic disorder:** "Exhibitionistic disorder" refers to a need—often accompanied by sexual gratification—to expose one's genitals to other individuals, both consensually and non-consensually. Exhibitionism with consenting adult participants does not qualify as a disorder unless the individual experiences significant distress or an impairment in functioning. A diagnosis is appropriate when the behavior—exposing one's genitals to unsuspecting individuals accompanied by sexual arousal—has occurred over an extended period of time.
- **Frotteuristic disorder:** Frotteuristic disorder is marked by strong sexual arousal associated with touching or rubbing against non-consenting individuals, often occurring in public settings such as buses or crowded spaces.

New Paraphilic Disorders

- **Otherwise specified paraphilic disorder:** This category is utilized when the paraphilia is not common enough to include its own diagnosis and falls outside of the eight primary paraphilic disorders; "examples include telephone scatologia (obscene phone calls), necrophilia (sexual activity with corpses), zoophilia, coprophilia (being aroused by being defecated upon or defecating on others), and urophilia (being aroused by being urinated upon or urinating on others)" (Beech et al., 2016).
- **Unspecified paraphilic disorder:** This category is applied when "clinically significant distress or impairment in social, occupational, or other important areas of functioning predominate but do not meet the full criteria for any of the disorders in the Paraphilic disorders diagnostic class" (American Psychiatric

Association, 2013). "More specifically, this category is used when a reason is not given for a specific paraphilic disorder criteria being specified because sufficient information may not be available" (Beech et al., 2016).

Many BDSM experts and kinksters alike hope for the day when BDSM is no longer associated with a mental health diagnosis. The *DSM* has conflated and continues to conflate sexual interests with criminal behaviors; and as this continues, so too will the discrimination and stigmatization of kinky people. However, it is important to note that it is incontrovertible that any sexual activity involving non-consenting adults or minors is highly problematic and constitutes a criminal act. In fact, as you will read in the following section, non-consensual sexual behavior is *always* a problem; and by definition, if someone is participating in non-consensual sexual behavior (or sexual behavior with a minor), they are not actually participating in kink—what they are participating in is abuse.

WHEN ARE SEXUAL BEHAVIORS A PROBLEM?

As seen above, three main themes can be considered when assessing whether sexual behavior is problematic: lack of consent, significant personal distress, and an impairment in functioning. While personal distress and impairment can be quite challenging to overcome, they often remain within the realm of the self, causing personal discomfort and emotional pain rather than causing harm to someone else. Each of these themes should be approached differently; however, it is safe to say that all non-consensual sexual behavior is a problem.

> The essence of nonconsensual sex is seen when one's behavior violates another person's freedom from sexual contact. It resides at the friction point between the sexual autonomy of two (or more) people. It happens when someone has sexual contact with a person who is unable to consent or when consent is obtained through coercion or force. It ranges on a continuum from various degrees of coarse sexual improprieties to low, medium, high, and lethal levels of sexual abuse and violence.
>
> Braun-Harvey & Vigorito, 2016

Even in cases where non-consent (i.e., consensual non-consent) is integrated into a D/s dynamic, it remains grounded in consent. Folks participating in any sexual behavior (including sexual behaviors that do not involve physical touch—that is, voyeurism and exhibitionism) without explicit prior permission (see Chapter 10 for a thorough description of this term) are engaging in highly problematic behavior, both ethically and legally.

While non-consent is straightforward (if there is no consent, it is a problem—period), when personal distress or impairment is involved, the issues immediately become more complex. Personal distress and impairment look different for everyone; thus, we must consider how those experiences manifest in someone's life. First, we need to consider what it means to be "significantly distressed." The *DSM-5* makes it clear that the personal distress someone feels regarding their paraphilia can not only be the result of societal stigma and disapproval (American Psychological Association, 2013). While this may seem like a helpful factor to consider, differentiating personal and societal-based distress is incredibly challenging as the impact of social stigma may not even be in our conscious awareness. It may take years of self-reflection to realize that something which feels personally distressing is actually a result of social stigma. Thus, it is important to consistently reevaluate our own sources of distress, as these will likely shift over time. So, while personal distress is an important factor to consider, when no non-consensual behaviors are occurring, the clearest indicator of problematic behavior may be the ways in which the desires or behaviors generate significant negative consequences in someone's life. Impairment can appear in various realms, including personal, occupational, financial, social, and relational. When a sexual behavior or desire begins to impact these various areas, it is time to take a much deeper look at it.

Out-of-Control Sexual Behavior

One particularly notable shift in understanding problematic sexual behavior was introduced to the therapeutic world when Doug Braun-Harvey and Michael Vigorito established the concept of "out-of-control sexual behavior" (OCSB). In 2016, their groundbreaking book *Treating Out of Control Sexual Behavior: Rethinking Sex Addiction* made the claim that OCSB is actually a "behavior problem within the normal range of sexual expression" rather than a clinical disorder (Braun-Harvey & Vigorito, 2016). The author's utilization of "out of control" refers to the subjective internal experiences of the individual—more specifically, a personal description of the various sensations, thoughts, perceptions, and emotions contributing to their sexual behavior problems. This new way of conceptualizing OCSB as a "sexual health problem in which consensual sexual urges, thoughts, or behaviors feel out of control" moves away from former modes of categorizing out-of-control behavior as "sexual addiction," "hyper-sexuality," or "dysregulated sexual behavior." "Phrases like 'sexual addiction' and 'compulsive sexual behavior' describe the sexual behavior problem using diagnostic labels that fuse a disease model with a description of a human behavior problem" (Braun-Harvey & Vigorito, 2016).

Braun-Harvey and Vigorito's model—drawn from descrip-tions of responsible sexual behavior by the Pan American Health Organization, the World Health Organization, and the World Association for Sexual Health—"operationalized the public health consensus on sexual health into a framework to mitigate the influence of proscriptive, disapproving, or stigmatizing sociocul-tural sexual values" (Braun-Harvey & Vigorito, 2016). This model has been utilized in particular for the treatment of OCSB in men; however, it appears to be a helpful overarching framework that can be applied to responsible sex in general, including among those who practice BDSM. "Integrating sexual health principles into the OCSB protocol [was] our attempt to remedy the justified fears of sociocultural norms that stigmatize the frequency or content of sexual urges, thoughts, and behaviors from overly influencing clin-ical intervention" (ibid).

The influence of fear and sociocultural norms on clinical inter-vention is a pervasive theme within the kink world, and using a framework such as that adapted by Braun-Harvey and Vigorito is an excellent way to assess when or whether sexual behavior is a problem. The six principles of responsible sexual behavior, as defined by Braun Harvey and Michael Vigorito, are as follows:

- **Consent**: a "voluntary cooperation" and the permission to reach sexual satisfaction and intimacy with oneself and willing part-ners (Wertheimer, 2003). Consent is a balance between one's autonomy to give clear, unambiguous consent for sex in com-bination with everyone's right to engage in sex with whom-ever [they choose] (Wertheimer, 2003). "Safe, consensual sex is a human right" (Swartzendruber & Zenilman, 2010) and the essential sexual health principle that makes mutually positive sexual interactions possible.

- **Nonexploitation**: Exploitation can be seen as leveraging one's power and control to receive sexual gratification from another person, which compromises that person's ability to consent. A person can increase the likelihood of non-exploitative sex when [they remain] highly motivated to ensure [they are] not taking unfair advantage to gain access to a sexual partner or sexual activity. Non-exploitative sex is likely when each person considers the risk of exploitation as it relates to the consent between partners, the potential for harm, and the mutual advantageousness for each person to enjoy the sexual situation (Wertheimer, 2003)

- **Protected from STIs and unintended pregnancy**:This Sexual Health principle is evident when those involved in the sexual activity are capable of protecting themselves and their partners from an STI (including HIV) and unintended or unwanted pregnancy period; this includes access to testing and medical care and scientifically accurate information regarding disease transmission, reproductive health, and contraception resources.

- **Honesty**: Sexual Health involves direct and open communication with oneself and one's partners. Self-honesty involves being open to sexual pleasure, experiences, and sexual education. Honesty is a crucial building block for sexual relations with others and is necessary for effective communication to uphold all of the sexual health principles. Honesty and sexual relationships vary based on relational factors and contexts and is not to be confused with complete transparency and unlimited candidness.

- **Shared Values**: Sexual relations between partners involve clarifying underlying motives, sexual standards, and the meaning of specific sexual acts for each person. This principle promotes conversations between sex partners to clarify their consent for sexual relations, discuss their sexual values, and articulate motivations for having sex.

- **Mutual Pleasure**:The mutual pleasure principle prioritizes the giving and receiving of pleasure.There are many ways for both giving and receiving sexual pleasure. Each moment of heightened pleasure can have many meanings that can change over time and with different partners.Valuing the pleasure of sex as a positive and life-enhancing aspect of sex is vital for ensuring Mutual pleasure. mutually pleasurable sexual activity invites clients to consider their bodily, erotic, and emotional sensualities for themselves and their partners.

Braun-Harvey & Vigorito, 2016

As well as reflecting on the concepts of impairment and personal distress, these principles paint a clear picture of what is and is not problematic behavior. There are several ways to engage in sexual and erotic exploration while maintaining a healthy and responsible approach. Adhering to the principles of responsible sexual behavior is a great starting point for participating in sexual activity from a consensual, informed, and mindful perspective.

If you feel that your sexual behavior may be problematic, please check out the list of additional resources for professional assistance.

ADDITIONAL RESOURCES

The Feminist Porn Book: The Politics of Producing Pleasure by Tristan Taormino, Constance Penley, Celine Parrenas Shimizu and Mireille Miller-Young (eds.)

Compulsive Sexual Behaviours by Silva Neves

Erotic Subjects and Outlaws: Sketching the Borders of Sexual Citizenship by Serena Petrella (ed.)

Sex Crimes: Research and Realities by Donna Vandiver and Jeremy Braithwaite

What Do We Know About the Effects of Pornography After Fifty Years of Academic Research? by Alan McKee, Katarina Litsou, et al.

9

ASSESSING RISK AND SAFETY
Stefani Goerlich

CONCEPTUALIZING RISK AND SAFETY

In 2010, in response to growing social concern about children "developing too quickly," an interdisciplinary team of researchers published *Healthy Sexual Development: A Multidisciplinary Framework for Research*, which identified 15 criteria necessary for healthy sexual development (McKee et al., 2010). The goal was to define what healthy sexual development looked like so that future researchers—as well as parents, pediatricians, and public policy advocates—would have a benchmark to measure both current behavior and future interventions against when determining what constituted "normal," healthy behavior and what was genuinely cause for concern. Their findings are useful not only in reassuring parents and informing sexual educators, but also for our purposes in conceptualizing what healthy kink engagement looks like. Let us look at each criterion through a kink-affirming lens:

- **Freedom from unwanted activity:** Kink should always be entered into enthusiastically, with a genuine sense of curiosity, desire, and/or play. Power exchange dynamics, in particular, must be mutually consensual. As Easton and Hardy have noted, one must have power in order to give it over to another (Easton & Hardy, 2001). If we do not feel able to say no to unwanted activity, this is not consensual kink—it is power theft. Healthy kink is predicated on everyone's right to refuse, opt out, or end a scene.

DOI: 10.4324/9781003312833-9

- **Sexual development should not be aggressive, coercive, or joyless:** It is a common misperception that BDSM and kink is meant to cause suffering to the submissive or bottoming person. The idea that sadomasochistic play hurts, that humiliation or degradation play evokes a sense of embarrassment, or that daily service represents an abnegation of self in favor of the other is a true but incomplete picture of how these scenes unfold. Kinky play should always meet the needs of the bottoming partner—whatever those needs may be. Whether the catharsis of emotional release or the high of an endorphin rush, the bottoming partner should NEVER walk away from a scene feeling sad, used, or upset. Even when the partners are enacting a scene that may be difficult in the moment, everyone involved should anticipate and be able to articulate the positive benefits this experience will have for them. If they cannot do so, it could be that this encounter is less about kink and more about coercive control or violence.

- **Education about sexual practices:** Many folks who experiment with BDSM are acting on knowledge and scenes they may have gleaned from pop culture depictions of kink. As we have discussed, these tend to be both inaccurate and incomplete. Therefore, it is vital that anyone curious about bringing elements of BDSM/kink into their lives and relationships take the time to seek out proper education about how to do so safely. This guidance is not limited to physical acts such as caning or tickling but should also include the emotional aspects of kink: how to negotiate a power exchange dynamic properly, what aftercare looks like when engaging in erotic humiliation, etc. There is no such thing as safe kink without informed kink. Knowing what educational resources are available for a broad spectrum of kink practices and being able to utilize or direct others to them is a crucial element of ethical BDSM.

- **Awareness of public/private boundaries:** It is possible to engage in BDSM in public. Dozens, if not hundreds, of kinky clubs and other spaces have been created for just this purpose. There are resorts, bed and breakfasts, cruises, and chatrooms where kinky people can interact and be present as their most authentic selves. Needless to say, these spaces do not include the grocery store, the public park, or the neighborhood block party. Particularly for those in power exchange relationships, and also for many fetishists, developing a sense of scale for their kink engagement—expanding their kinky nature at home and contracting to be a bit more circumspect in public—is a core aspect of their BDSM learning curve. Many new practitioners—and even passionate, experienced players—take great pride in their kinky natures and want to be able to express that aspect of themselves without shame or stigma. However, we must always be aware of the fact that others may not consent to be a part of our scene (as watchers or bystanders), and that we must respect social norms and boundaries—even if we feel like it should be perfectly acceptable to walk our fully clothed spouse through the zoo on a collar and leash.

- **An understanding of consent:** Studies have shown that the BDSM community likely has a stronger consent culture than the mainstream, simply because of the emphasis placed on negotiation and boundary setting between partners. Having a nuanced view of consent and understanding the various forms that consent can and should take—including physical consent, emotional consent, informed consent, evolving consent, withdrawing consent, and the spectrum of consent violations—is a critical part of ethical kink. In particular, this is the case when exploring scenarios in which one person will be holding authority over or engaging in rougher physical play with another.

- **An understanding of safety:** Because many BDSM practices (even those that involve no physical or sexual contact) carry a degree of risk, an understanding of safety is emphasized not only as a healthy part of sexuality but as a necessary foundation for the healthy practice of kink. As we will learn later on in this chapter, the kink community has conceptualized several ways to describe this expectation over the years and safe engagement—not only with one's partners but also with oneself—remains a core element of what it means to be an ethical kinkster.

- **Self-acceptance:** Internalized guilt and shame for falling outside of the socially prescribed "Charmed Circle" plagues gender, sexuality, and relationship minorities of all stripes. When not addressed, this can manifest as pathologization of one's desires (e.g., describing oneself as "addicted"); abstinence from relationships and experiences that would otherwise be affirming and pleasurable; or even the use of elements of BDSM such as humiliation/degradation to reinforce one's sense of brokenness.

A strong grounding in pleasure equity and intimate justice, an openminded critique of behavioral "addiction" models, and psychoeducation about the prevalence of BDSM practices within the general population can be transformative for people who otherwise struggle to recognize themselves as healthy and worthy people and partners. BDSM should always be explored from a place of self-love and affirmation. When it becomes an expression of self-loathing, we must pause to address the underlying internal struggles that this represents.

- **Acceptance that sex can be pleasurable:** To continue the point above, healthy kink requires that everyone involved recognize that their experiences can (and should) be pleasurable. Admittedly, "pleasure" can take many forms! The masochist derives intense pleasure from experiencing sensations that may not otherwise be described as pleasant. When we are reflecting on the idea of healthy sexual development within the context of BDSM, we must be careful not to conflate the two. Oftentimes, isolated elements of BDSM expression may be unpleasant, but the cumulative experience of a given scene or relationship should be pleasurable for those involved. One of the factors that differentiates consensual kink from intimate partner violence is the understanding that both partners should experience positive outcomes from whatever experience they have negotiated. When we see patterns of belief that require one partner to be deprived of pleasure entirely while the other exclusively benefits, we should think critically about whether this represents a healthy expression of kink for those involved.
- **Sexual agency:** BDSM engagement of any form should always be entered into consensually by those involved. Whether we are exploring the exchange of control, the exchange of authority, or the exchange of sensation, the key word is "exchange." Everyone involved should feel safe asking for what they want and need, setting boundaries for their bodies and relationships, and iterating their relationship dynamics over time. It is a common misstatement that "the submissive holds all the power in the relationship" when it comes to kink; but the converse is also true—no one should ever feel disempowered or unwillingly constrained within a kink dynamic.
- **Relationship skills:** Communication, frustration tolerance, and conflict management are core skills for any relationship,

kinky or otherwise. Often, we fall into patterns of focusing on BDSM skills—safe rope technique; protecting the kidneys from floggers—and fail to engage in the same level of general relationship skill-building. Before anyone engages in kinky play with their partner or an enthusiastic friend, they should also be developing their emotional intelligence muscles, their empathy, their non-verbal communication skills, and their ability to self-regulate when personalities or desires inevitably clash.

- **Open communication:** There are many dominant personalities who worry that if they allow themselves to be vulnerable, to talk about their needs, to ask their partners for something, they are somehow undermining their own authority. Likewise, many submissive folks worry that if they set a boundary, if they express a desire, if they ask for more or less in their relationship, they are somehow failing to "properly" serve and are thus not submitting "enough." Challenging these internal fears and reminding ourselves that open and ongoing communication is a necessary element not only for our own sexual and relational health but for our partner's as well can inspire us to re-envision these moments as opportunities to deepen our service to heighten our protection of our partners and our relationship.
- **Lifelong learning:** There will never be a time when we have finished learning about sexuality, relationships, or BDSM/kink. Whether we are exploring the ways in which our safety practices need to evolve as our bodies age or how technology can both protect us and expose us to risk, there will always be more to learn. We should maintain a learner's mindset, recognizing that these skills can always evolve no matter how highly skilled we may be. It is a hallmark of sexual health.
- **Resilience:** BDSM and other kinky play often test the endurance of participants. This might mean physical endurance. Often, it takes the form of emotional fortitude. Resilience—the ability to recover from setbacks and rebound from difficulty—is a necessary skill. Where one forms agreements, it is possible for these agreements to be violated. We accept the energy drain associated with challenging tasks when we take them on. And where we form strong, trusting bonds, we must be prepared that these bonds may end. This is the nature of human connection and relationships; and it is magnified when we add elements of control, authority, and sensation exchange. Fortitude, tolerance, and self-care are the hallmarks of the resilient kinkster.

- **Understanding parental and social values:** Even within a 27/4 dynamic between partners who are quite open and shame-free about their kink identities, healthy kink will inevitably have some necessary limits. In the same way that most parents do not discuss their preferred sexual position or frequency of inter-course with their children, kinky parents are likely to self-censor or scale back aspects of their relationship in ways they may not have had to prior to parenting. For some kinksters, this can feel frustrating—particularly when relational behaviors (e.g., kneeling or the use of honorifics) that are not overtly sexual must be scaled back to accommodate the presence of their children in the household. Likewise, there are situations and locations socially where overt BDSM is not ethical. The clichéd example of the Dom walking her slave through the grocery store on a leash comes to mind. Ethical kink requires a consideration of the context in which it occurs and the consent of those who may be present. Finding ways to maintain authentic connections with their partners while also fulfilling social and parental roles that may feel stifling or constraining can be a source of frustration for some kinky clients. Clients who are unwilling or unable to adjust their kink presentation/behavior to a given social setting or household role may benefit from psychoeducation on sex-positive boundary setting and consent.
- **Competence in mediated sexuality:** The ability to differ-entiate the performative nature of BDSM as it is portrayed in popular culture and erotica from the ways in which BDSM and kink typically present in everyday life is a core skill for anyone wanting to incorporate elements of BDSM/kink into their lives and relationships. Kinky people in pop culture are often portrayed as one of two archetypes: either a danger to others or the butt of a joke. As a result, it is difficult for kinky people to find positive portrayals of everyday BDSM that make them feel validated and seen. At the opposite end of the spectrum, pornography often presents a much more extreme—even dark—depiction of kink that can also leave viewers feeling unrepresented. Differentiating between the exaggerated fantasies of porn, the stigmatizing por-trayals of pop culture, and their own lived reality of life as a BDSM practitioner can be a source of minority stress and mar-ginalization for some clients; and a source of misinformation and miseducation for others.

KINK-AFFIRMING RISK ASSESSMENT

Kink-affirming risk assessment is one of the most difficult skills to learn as a clinician. The experience of anti-kink stigma, our own potential for bias toward some forms of kink expression, and the very real need to balance our ethical obligations with our clients' need for us to hold space for their darkest desires can make the idea of trying to assess risk and safety from a kink-affirming perspective feel overwhelming, if not impossible. Being able to hold space for honest and authentic conversations about not only the potential benefits of BDSM/kink for our clients but also the very real potential for harm can be a frightening prospect. This fear exists on both sides of the treatment room and can result in our clients strategically withholding information or downplaying the true nature of their BDSM/kink practices or power exchange dynamics until we have demonstrated our trustworthiness and ability to meet their authentic selves without judgment. "Maintaining confidentiality and therapeutic boundaries is crucial for creating a safe environment. Furthermore, the therapist's ability to pass clients' tests and deactivate their defenses is key to enabling clients to safely disclose and explore potentially dangerous material" (Podolan & Gelo, 2023). There are four qualities necessary for effective kink-affirming risk and safety assessment—and, one might argue, effective therapy in general.

Autonomy and Agency

Fostering a client's sense of personal agency and autonomy when assessing them for risk and safety is a critical component in kink-affirming clinical practice. A therapeutic environment that prioritizes the individual's wellbeing while respecting their inherent rights and choices shows them that we recognize that they are capable of making well-reasoned, informed decisions about their personal safety, relationships, and mental health. When we center agency and autonomy in our safety planning and risk assessment processes, clinicians build a foundation of trust, empower their clients, and model how to discuss and negotiate risk-management strategies—an important skill for our kinky clients outside of the treatment room as well.

Kink-affirming therapy acknowledges that the client is the expert on their own life, experiences, values, and desires. No matter how deep the clinician's knowledge of BDSM cultures, practices, or skills might be, their knowledge will never surpass that of each individual client. The process of centering client agency and autonomy involves actively listening to their specific narrative, understanding their unique BDSM/kink context, and appreciating the ways in which their experiences with and perspectives on BDSM/kink might vary from those of other clients or the clinician themselves. Centering the client's specific lived experiences—particularly when assessing risk and safety planning—fosters a therapeutic alliance based on trust, openness, mutual respect, and informed consent. Informed consent lies at the heart of both ethical therapy and ethical BDSM/kink. Ensuring that our clients are actively involved in decision-making processes related to their treatment is one of the most basic expectations of therapeutic practice. Within kink-affirming practice, informed consent should ideally be a dynamic process that mirrors the negotiation and renegotiation ethos of the BDSM community and allows clients to make choices based on their evolving needs and preferences.

For some clients who have a history of trauma, disrupted attachment, or consent violations, risk and safety conversations can feel retraumatizing. When someone who has had their autonomy violated in the past experiences a relationship that prioritizes their agency and autonomy, the treatment room can become a healing space—even when difficult conversations happen there.

> A client's sense of safety is predictive of the treatment outcome. More specifically, clients' early feeling of safety predicts subsequent treatment improvement, with early alliance mediating this relationship. Client-rated session safety is associated with session positivity, smoothness, and depth, as well as with the therapeutic bond, confident collaboration, and overall alliance.
>
> Podolan & Gelo, 2023

By allowing clients to assert control over their therapeutic journey and (concurrently) the process of assessing their degree of risk and formulating a safety strategy, the clinician creates a safe and validating atmosphere, minimizes the risk of re-enacting past traumas, and fosters a sense of security within the therapeutic relationship.

Client-Centered

One of the core values of person-centered therapy is the notion that our clients are making the best choices they can for themselves with the information and resources available to them at the time. This is especially true when it comes to their understanding of and tolerance for risk and safety—physical, emotional, or relational. "Persons are realizing their potentialities and protecting themselves as best they can at any given time and under the internal and external circumstances that exist at that time" (Borzarth, 2024). Working together with clients, we can help them create their own personal risk framework, identify potential dangers within that framework, and devise strategies to mitigate or prevent them by centering the client's expertise and their unique insights into their own lives. We can ask good questions and offer psychoeducational and learning resources; but we cannot make choices *for* our clients because they are far more likely to develop meaningful safety measures for themselves than we are as outside observers—even kink-competent outside observers. And when they operate from a place of empowered agency, they are far more likely to succeed in implementing these strategies consistently as well.

One happy side-effect of centering our clients' agency and autonomy is that it leads to more effective safety plans. When clients feel their choices and preferences are honored (even when they are choosing to engage in behaviors or relationship dynamics that the clinician might be personally uncomfortable with or concerned about), they are more likely to feel a sense of ownership over their therapy experience and their behavioral/relational choices outside of the treatment room (Peasant, 2014). An empowered client can understand the necessary process of risk and safety assessment as an opportunity for collaboration and co-learning with their therapist rather than as a judgment made about them personally. This collaborative mindset fosters a sense of personal responsibility for understanding and managing risk, and enhances the client's ability to make the decisions that are best for them and actively contribute to their own safety. Ultimately, prioritizing agency and autonomy contributes to a kink-affirming, client-centered approach that respects the dignity and uniqueness of each individual on their journey toward authenticity and self-discovery.

Non-Judgmental

Most clinicians believe that they are capable of maintaining a neutral affect and a non-biased perspective to their work with clients. This is a central element of training as a psychotherapist and an ideal that clinicians of all disciplines are taught to aspire to. For many kink-affirming therapists, the idea of being kink-affirming is understood as a corrective against the anti-kink stigma that so many of our clients experience in other settings or with other providers. We tend to assume that being kink-affirming is the same as being nonjudgmental because we are not judging our clients' alternative relationship dynamics or sensory desires. However, even a positive bias toward BDSM/kink is a bias. All biases carry some clinical risk—the risk of "romancing the kink," to give one example (Goerlich, 2020). We could consider this positive regard for BDSM/kink to be an example of the intersubjective field at work, especially if the clinician is themselves kink identified. "An intersubjective field is created by the interplay between the subjective inner worlds of the patient and therapist" (Frayn, 1990). In this context of risk assessment, this inner world is the clinician's own understanding of what safe and ethical BDSM/kink "should" look like versus what their client might envision for themselves.

> The intersubjective field reflects personality elements and histories brought to therapeutic encounters separately by therapists and patients that join to create new kinds of therapeutic relationships. This concept acknowledges that therapists' subjectivity is requisite and undoubtedly provides key avenues for understanding patients—but it is subjective.
>
> Yager et al., 2021

Kinky or not, therapists may struggle with their own emotional reactions to clients' disclosures—especially when it comes to edgier forms of play, such as intensive sadomasochism, degradation/humiliation play, or race play. It can be challenging to set aside personal judgments or emotional responses triggered by clients' stories, especially when they involve situations that may feel like moral or ethical dilemmas to the listener. Being aware of our impulse to label a client's behavior as not "real" BDSM/kink because it does not align with our own preferred style of power exchange or understanding of safety should be an ongoing part of the process of self-regulation during sessions with kinky clients. Even within the already stigmatized BDSM community, there are subcommunities that experience marginalization from their kinky peers. Clients whose relationship dynamics or erotic desires are spurned even within the wider world of BDSM may be grappling with feelings of isolation and shame that are compounded by microaggressions or rejection in spaces that should feel safe for erotic outsiders. A non-judgmental therapist who can set aside their own notions of what BDSM/kink "should" look like and encourage them to express their own understandings of risk, safety, ethics, etc. openly is a therapist who will help to foster a more honest and authentic therapeutic process. When clients feel accepted and understood—in therapy if nowhere else on Earth—they are more likely to share their innermost thoughts and emotions, contributing to a deeper exploration of their concerns.

Curious

Curiosity is a motivational tool that plays a crucial role in building trust and rapport within the therapeutic relationship. "Compassion and curiosity remain the best tools therapists can use in their efforts to serve their patients" (Lefevre, 2012). Understanding and supporting our clients and affirming their humanity and dignity, even when they share fantasies and desires that trigger discomfort or concern in the clinician, is the most powerful work of kink-affirming therapy. Our ability to remain curious in such moments, rather than moving into a place of alarm or intervention, fosters empathy, encourages exploration, and ultimately results in more positive therapeutic outcomes (ibid).

When faced with worrisome disclosures that activate our internal professional "alarm bells," curiosity encourages therapists to set aside preconceived notions of what risk and safety look like and hold space for the client's own understanding of their stories and experiences. Most kink-affirming therapists are quite good at avoiding pathologizing perspectives on BDSM, of course. Nevertheless, we still operate within the intersubjective fields that we have built with each client and may still experience an impulse to explain, correct, or intervene (Goerlich, 2023). A curious therapist will notice their desire to act and choose instead to ask questions that help them understand the context, motivations, and underlying emotions behind the client's disclosures. Curiosity allows us to maintain our non-judgmental, client-centered perspective. By prioritizing the individual's own understanding of their identity, desires, relationships, and experiences, we avoid imposing our own personal values, beliefs, and "shoulds" upon them. We allow them the space to feel heard and validated rather than challenged or corrected—even when discussing topics that may be considered problematic or high-risk (Hannigan, 2023).

Curiosity allows us to explore potential alternatives without assigning value to the alternatives and to problem-solve without the client feeling they are being identified as problematic. It allows us to hold space for the idea of "safe uncertainty . . . an approach which focuses on safety but takes into account changing information, different perspectives and acknowledges that certainty may not be achievable" (Phillips et al., 2022). Instead of either confronting or avoiding difficult topics, kink-affirming therapists can use curiosity to lean into this uncertainty and encourage deeper exploration that can lead the client to insights that contribute toward the co-creation of effective interventions and strategies for addressing the concerns that first brought them to counseling.

COMMUNITY FRAMEWORKS

Over the last 50 years or so, the BDSM/kink community has developed a variety of models that kinky people can use to help them understand, name, evaluate, and prioritize the variables within their own personal risk framework. Prior to the 1970s, the idea of BDSM/kink as something that could be "safe" was almost laughable. Deeply embedded cultural gender norms, virulent homophobia, stringent censorship laws, and the pervasive risk of either criminal or psychiatric institutionalization if kinky people were outed as "deviants" effectively negated any hope of risk-free exploration. This began to change with the arrival of the AIDS crisis. In the earliest days of the AIDS crisis, anti-kink bias redoubled.

> In North America and the UK, the first people affected by AIDS were leathermen. For this reason, leathermen often faced stigma within the lesbian and gay communities that reinforced pre-existing prejudices against the fetish communities. For example, BDSM and fisting (using the fist for anal sex) were labeled as particularly dangerous, even in the absence of scientific evidence.
>
> Slagstad, 2023

Within a few years, however, as awareness of how the virus was spread grew, activists began to propose that BDSM could actually serve as a HIV harm reduction/mitigation strategy (Lowrey, 2004), since kinky play creates opportunities for erotic intimacy and sensory expression that do not require nudity—or even direct physical contact—to be mutually satisfying. Amid this debate and the growing awareness of physical (rather than interpersonal, social, or legal) danger, the first BDSM safety model was named.

SSC

In 1983, the founding members of the Gay Male S/M Activists (GMSMA) drafted their statement of identity and purpose. Written by slave david stein (sic), it began: "GMSMA is a not-for-profit organization of gay males in the New York City area who are seriously interested in safe, sane, and consensual S/M" (Stein, 2000). Riffing on a phrase used to encourage responsible fireworks on Independence Day, the GMSMA initially envisioned "safe, sane, and consensual" (SSC) as a rebuttal to the stigma described above.

> We were trying to draw a line between what is clearly defensible, in terms of both social structures and personal well-being and what is either indefensible or at least very questionable. It was a conscious, deliberate attempt to shift the debate onto grounds we thought we could win, instead of having to keep proving we weren't serial killers, spouse beaters, and child abusers.
>
> Ibid

SSC has been criticized as reductionist, ableist, and overly expansive by many over the years—critiques that stein acknowledged and wrote about during his life; but it did represent a shift in the BDSM community's relationship to the mainstream. No longer were kinky people willing to be defined by outsiders, from their vanilla peers in the queer liberation movement to the suburban cops entrapping them in honeypots; they were taking the lead in defining what ethical kink should look like—and that makes this simple, three-word phrase a revolutionary statement and one that grew in popular usage throughout the 1980s and early 1990s.

RACK

With the rise of the internet age, bulletin board services and email listservs skyrocketed in popularity among marginalized people of all kinds, and BDSM practitioners around the world began to find each other and build communities in online spaces. One of the many conversations that this new technology facilitated was allowing critics of the SSC model to find each other and share their ideas without needing to be located in major geographic centers such as New York or San Francisco. Now, a lesbian activist in Minnesota could find a HIV/AIDS educator in Germany and share their thoughts and opinions about how safe and ethical kink should be defined. On November 25, 1999, Gary Switch posted the following on the TES-Friends list, which he requested be reproduced in whole:

I proposed RACK (Risk-Aware, Consensual Kink) as an alternative. Here's my motivation:

Nothing's perfectly safe. Crossing the street isn't perfectly safe. Remember that it's technically called "safer sex," not "safe sex." If we want to limit BDSM to what's safe, we can't do anything more extreme than flogging somebody with a wet noodle. Mountain climbers don't call their sport safe, for the simple reason that it isn't; risk is an essential part of the thrill. They handle it by identifying and minimizing the risk through study, training, technique, and practice. I believe that this approach will work better for us leatherfolk than claiming that what we do is safe. We want to foster the notion that we develop expertise, that to do what we do properly takes skill developed through a similar process of education, training, and practice.

Negotiation cannot be valid without foreknowledge of the possible risks involved in the activity being negotiated. "Risk-aware" means that both parties to a negotiation have studied the proposed activities, are informed about the risks involved, and agree how they intend to handle them. Hence "risk-aware" instead of "safe."

The "sane" part of SSC is very subjective. Who's making the call? Person A might think fisting is insane; persons B and C might enjoy it very much. "Sane" always reminds me of Pat Paulsen's campaign slogan from the old Smothers Brothers show: "Vote for Paulsen; he's not insane!" If you go around constantly reassuring folks that you're not crazy, they'll start to wonder.

I've heard "sane" interpreted as: "able to distinguish fantasy from reality" and "not intoxicated," which are both perfectly valid, though the latter is similar to the above—you don't go around constantly reassuring folks that you're not drunk, either.

"Consensual" is the crux, implying negotiation which implies being able to distinguish fantasy from reality, as well as dealing responsibly with risk factors. If you don't know the risk factors, if you don't know what will happen in reality, then you don't know what you're consenting to. Meaningful negotiation must always take place on the common ground of consensus reality.

The "kink" part went in to make a snappy acronym and because SSC doesn't tell you what you should be SSC about. Safe, Sane, and Consensual trout fishing? Alluding to the rack, an archetypal torture instrument, has been criticized, but to me it signifies our transformation of atrocity into ecstasy, and admits that though we may enjoy some dark fantasies, we realize them harmlessly.

RACK is admittedly more confrontational than SSC. It's defiant, the same way the GLBT community uses "queer." RACK allows us the freedom to have non-PC fantasies. Don't a lot of us enjoy non-consensual fantasies, either from the top side or the bottom side? We enjoy them in our literature; we may very well enjoy them while we play. But we act them out responsibly and consensually.

Switch, 2018

Today, RACK has become the predominant risk assessment model used within the BDSM community and those who support it. However, it does have successors that build on the pragmatic foundation that Switch created.

FRIES

Planned Parenthood of America introduced the FRIES model of consent, which was quickly adopted by sexual health activists ranging from BDSM/kink educators to Hollywood intimacy coordinators and beyond. FRIES stands for: "Freely given," "Reversible," "Informed," "Enthusiastic," "Specific."

While not specific to BDSM, the FRIES model offers a user-friendly mnemonic to remember the elements of ethical negotiation and play. The element of informed consent is present in both RACK (risk awareness is not possible without information about what risks are possible) and FRIES; however, FRIES expands the "erotic information map" even further by requiring specificity. Within the FRIES model, it is not sufficient to say, "I consent to an impact scene." We must break down what that means into specific elements—for example:

I consent to a "thuddy"-feeling impact scene with you using a thick flogger or your open palm. I am even open to a closed fist, but only if you strike my buttocks where I'll get the most "thud." I do not enjoy stinging sensations, so I do not consent to being struck with a bamboo cane or single-tail whip.

Emphasizing freely given and enthusiastic also connects FRIES to the earlier SSC model, which defined "sanity" in part as being neither coerced nor given while under the influence of substances. Within the sex education space, FRIES has become quite popular—likely due to its origins within the Planned Parenthood organization—and has served as a nice addition to the kink community's RACK model.

4Cs

In 2014, a new BDSM-specific negotiation framework was proposed by Dr. D.J. Williams and the Center for Positive Sexuality, which encompasses four specific dimensions: consent, communication, caring, and caution. This 4Cs model was designed to address the limitations already acknowledged within the SSC model and problems that Williams et al. identified within the RACK framework. Both SSC and RACK center some notion of safety—either explicitly (as in SSC) or implicitly (as something that kinksters need to be "aware" of in RACK). The 4Cs model replaces this with the notion of caution.

> We have observed that many BDSM participants seem to defer, knowingly or not, to somewhat strict medical discourses concerning discussions of risk and safety. In this sense, RACK seems preferable to SSC, yet we still realize that SSC has become more restrictive and perhaps codified than was originally intended . . . Our preference of the word caution is an acknowledgment of longstanding politics concerning bodies and sexuality, and allows for a wide range of meanings and motivations for engaging in various possible forms of BDSM.
>
> Williams et al., 2014

One of the key contributions that the 4Cs model offers to our understanding of both risk and safety is the concept of consent. Williams et al. acknowledge that for many, their BDSM play includes role-played coercion, consensual non-consent (both sexual and in terms of rules and protocols), and other gradations that can make kinky consent more complicated than it might appear on the surface. The 4Cs model acknowledges three specific layers of consent:

- **Surface consent:** The binary, yes-or-no consent that comes to most people's minds when thinking about the topic.
- **Scene consent:** The more detailed, structured negotiation process that BDSM practitioners engage in prior to engaging in kinky play together, including the mechanism by which the parties can communicate that they are withdrawing their consent.

- **Deep consent:** "Here we are talking about something beyond just a bottom's ability to use a safeword or gesture. For instance, when a bottom is crying and sobbing and in obvious distress and perhaps full into some kind of subspace—but has not yet been called 'red'—we might wonder to what extent the scene is affecting the thinking of the bottom and affecting the bottom's mental capacity to yell out 'red' or to engage in cognitive consent at all? In addition, even if the bottom is still able to think, the bottom may not actually know whether he or she is consenting. In such cases, it seems like the question of consent is something that almost has to be considered after the fact. As the bottom plays back the scene in the hours and days and weeks that follow, he or she might come to some kind of conclusion: 'I consented' or 'no I didn't' or perhaps 'I guess I just don't know.' In addition, it is important to be aware that aftercare and later conversations (especially between the top and bottom) may actually change the bottom's interpretation of a scene and his or her consequent view of consent" (ibid).

Deep consent can occur within scenes that meet the FRIES and RACK criteria, but may still feel unsettling or confusing to the partners afterward. Because it is so often assessed (or even revoked) retrospectively, our understanding of deep consent is critical to our understanding of how power can be abused or misused within BDSM play, even when one or both parties believe in the moment that they have given and received full consent.

4Ps

One way the ambiguity discussed above can be evaluated after the fact is through the 4Ps model. Developed by co-author Stefani Goerlich as an attempt to integrate her work as a forensic social worker specializing in sexual violence with her training as a kink-affirming sex therapist, the 4Ps model was first published in a special 2024 edition of the *Journal of Couple and Family Psychoanalysis*. Goerlich developed the 4Ps model to address the resistance many of her kink-identified survivor clients expressed toward more traditional "power and control" frameworks of intimate partner violence. She observed that for survivors in power exchange dynamics, the concept of one partner holding power over another could be difficult to conceptualize as a negative thing. To address this legitimate relationship difference while still acknowledging that abuse is possible within BDSM relationships, and that the language of BDSM can be used to mask abuse in other relationships, she began to ask her clients to assess their sense of personal power and control within their relationship using four specific tiers:

- **Pleasure:** Mutually satisfying, desired, and enjoyable encounters of all kinds—sexual, relational, sensory, or beyond. These can include elements of power or sensory exchange that may mirror non-consensual scenarios or evoke a counter-transference reaction in the clinician, but are defined by the pleasure they evoke for all involved.
- **Performance:** Sexual and relational experiences that are less desired at first, which are entered into by the client with the expectation that they may experience reactive desire or find other enjoyable elements once the encounter begins. These moments are freely entered into and consensual but may not be experienced as deeply pleasurable.
- **Persuasion:** Any encounter that the client agrees to engage in due to feeling pressured, nagged, guilted, or otherwise persuaded to participate in that they would not otherwise choose for themselves. This can range from passive-aggressive comments and emotional manipulation to threats of outing and other more aggressive verbal threats. Encounters motivated by persuasion are not experienced as pleasurable or reactively desired by the client and may be described as ambiguously consensual.
- **Power theft:** Power theft occurs in any scenario where the client feels that their boundaries have been violated, their limits disrespected, or their needs unmet. The term "power theft" can be more relatable for kinky survivors. Goerlich writes:"[T]here is no power exchange where one has no power to give" (Goerlich, 2024). Introducing "power theft" into the client's understanding of their relationship can be a helpful way to hold space for power exchange while also acknowledging that not all power taken by one partner in a relationship is consensually given by the other.

RISK ASSESSMENT CHECKLIST

It is both possible and necessary to be both kink-affirming and mindful of the potential for risk that arises from many kinds of behavior—both intimate and otherwise. As with food, exercise, thrill-seeking, and substance use, it is possible for any highly sensory experience to be taken to an unhealthy extreme. It is not kink-shaming to be aware of the potential risks that exist within BDSM and to work to assess various kink behaviors and their associated risk potentials. Whether we are a clinician considering a formal paraphilia diagnosis (something that should be avoided wherever possible—see Chapter Ten for more guidance) or simply engaging in active self-reflection to develop our own personal risk tolerance profile, the questions that follow can be used as framework for conceptualizing potential areas of concern to address in your personal kink practice, your client's reported behavior, or both.

- **Origins:**
  - **Age of first interest:** How old were you the first time you noticed an interest/feeling that you would, later in adulthood, describe as kinky?
  - **Age of first exposure:** How old were you the first time that you were exposed to media or experiences that you would label as kinky?
  - **Age of first engagement:** How old were you the first time you participated in activities you would label as kinky?
  - **Consent in first exposure/engagement:** Were these early experiences (exposure, engagement) consensual? Did they occur within a context that felt fun, safe, and pleasurable for you?
- **Safety:**
  - **Ongoing affirmative consent:** When you engage in kink, how do you give/receive/reconfirm consent throughout the scene?
  - **Safety planning/safe word:** What safety planning/research do you do before a scene? Do you use a safe word? Do you keep safety or first aid equipment on-hand?
  - **Risk/history of serious injury:** Do you engage in play that is high risk (e.g., breath play) or likely to result in injury (e.g., heavy impact, knife play)? Do you have a history of giving or receiving injury requiring medical treatment during kink play?
  - **Aftercare:** What does aftercare look like for you? Do all parties (top and bottom) receive aftercare? Can aftercare be withheld or denied?

- **Family history:**

  - **History of abuse or trauma:** Do you have a history of physical, sexual, or emotional abuse? Have you experienced other traumas outside of your family of origin? (NOTE: Kink and trauma are NOT correlated. Kinky people report rates of trauma at the same rate as their vanilla peers. This information is useful in understanding how we conceptualize our/their kinky practices and identities, but is not typically relevant to a clinical assessment of their kink engagement.)

  - **Attachment:** How do you describe your relationships with your family of origin? How does your attachment style impact your relationship engagement with partners?

  - **Relationships today:** Do you have supportive relationships with your family of origin today? If not, how does this impact your sense of self and adult life?

- **Daily experiences:**

  - **Interference with activities of daily living/instrumental activities of daily living:** Do you struggle with activities of daily living (ADLs)/instrumental activities of daily living (IADLs)? If so, does your kink play serve as a supportive factor in this area or could it be a source of friction/resistance to ADLs/IADLs?

  - **Dissociation or disorientation:** Do you experience moments of disorientation (an inability to correctly gauge the current time, place, one's role and one's identity) (Victoria

Activities for Daily Living	*Instrumental Activities of Daily Living*
• Ambulation/movement	• Caring for others
• Dressing	• Caring for pets
• Feeding	• Childrearing
• Bathing/showering	• Shopping/errands
• Personal hygiene	• Communication management
• Toileting	• Driving/community mobility
	• Financial management
	• Health management/maintenance
	• Home care/management
	• Meal preparation and clean-up
	• Spiritual engagement (if any)
	• Safety end emergency response

Source: Lyon, 2023

Department of Health, 2023) or dissociation (a mental process where a person disconnects from their thoughts, feelings, memories, or sense of identity) (Schnider, 2012)? Do these experiences occur spontaneously or are they triggered by an activating event? Do you engage in BDSM play during these moments?

- **Blurred boundaries:** Do you engage in (or feel pressure to engage in) BDSM play at times or in places that would be inappropriate, such as at work? Are you able to "step in and out of role" with your partners? Are you able to set clear boundaries around your sexual/relational self, your desires, your needs, your limits?
- **Compulsive behaviors:** Do you engage in behaviors that you do not feel able to control? Do you feel capable of leaving a situation or ending a scene if you wish to? Do you feel impulsive in your decision-making? Do you feel capable of saying no to your play partners or yourself?

- **Social supports:**

  - **Spouse/partner reactions:** Do you feel that you can share your authentic self and desires with your partner? Do you feel supported by your partner? Are you able to explore your needs and desires together with your partner?
  - **Friends/family acceptance:** Do you have friends and/ or family who understand and affirm your kink identity? Do you feel capable of being your authentic self around the people who are important to you?
  - **Messages from faith community (if any):** Are you connected to a faith/spiritual community? What is your understanding of sexuality, intimacy, and relationships from this perspective? What are your views on sin and the body? How do these inform your understanding of and relationship to kink?
  - **Connections to kink community:** Do you live in an area with a thriving kink community? Can you access opportunities for socialization, learning, and support? If not, do you maintain a presence on kinky social media or otherwise find supportive outlets? Can you access community education regarding specific kink practices if needed/desired?

- **Stressors:**

  - **Personal distress:** Do you experience guilt about your kinky play or relationships? Do you feel shame about your kink identity or desires? Do you wish you could change yourself or be "vanilla"?
  - **Disrupted relationships:** Have you experienced rejection or stigma within your relationships due to your kink identities? Does kink play get in the way of parenting or partnerships? Are you diverting household resources/moneys in order to engage in your sexual/intimate activities?
  - **Interference with work:** Are you engaging in kink behaviors in the workplace or while on work time? Have you taken significant time off work in order to engage in kink play? Has your employer disciplined you for inappropriate computer usage, wardrobe, or behavior?
  - **Illegal activities:** Regardless of whether others have caught you, have you engaged in non-consensual conduct such as voyeurism, exhibitionism, or unwanted touching of others? Have you engaged in theft in order to acquire desired fetish objects? Have you used illegal drugs as a part of your sexual/intimate behaviors? Are you misappropriating funds (e.g., from employers, children's savings, family members) in order to afford your sexual/intimate behaviors?

The above should be used as a jumping-off point for assessing the likelihood of risk related to our behavior (across a wide spectrum of behaviors, both sexual and non) and our own responsibility to understand and adjust these behaviors to mitigate potential harm effectively. The concerns listed above are not exclusive to people who enjoy BDSM and kink—all of the above can and do occur without the presence of kink or BDSM interest. This section should be viewed as an example of risk assessment that is framed to support an exploration of risk for kinky people; however, it is just as useful for folks grappling with video game usage, pornography consumption, sports betting, or excessive exercise, to name just a few areas of passionate interest that can, without modulation, veer into problematic territory. The questions are the start of a conversation, not a binary analysis of safe versus harmful. These conversations should always occur with the foundational understanding that kink itself is NEVER the risk factor.

ADDITIONAL RESOURCES

Assessing and Managing Problematic Sexual Interests: A Practitioner's Guide by Geraldine Akerman and Derek Perkins (eds.)

Power: A User's Guide by Julie Diamond

Sadomasochism in Everyday Life: The Dynamics of Power and Powerlessness by Lynn S. Chancer

Boundaries: When to Say Yes, How to Say No to Take Control of Your Life by Henry Cloud and John Townsend

SexSmart: How Your Childhood Shaped Your Sexual Life and What to Do About It by Aline P. Zoldbrod

BEST PRACTICES FOR WORKING WITH KINKY CLIENTS

Elyssa Helfer

POWER AND CONTROL IN THE TREATMENT ROOM

Whether consciously or unconsciously, power dynamics are at play within every relationship we have. From our relationships with family members to those with work associates, community leaders and more, we are embedded in a system where power dynamics permeate all areas of life. While it certainly may be true that folks within a romantic or sexual dynamic are striving for an intentional way of relating—whether egalitarian or consensually hierarchical—when it comes to professional contexts, it may be harder to land on an equal balance where inherent power dynamics are present. Particularly within the realm of psychotherapy, a variety of power-related issues can arise; some of these we can work to change, but others are so deeply embedded in the system that they may be hard to break free from. It is critical for mental health providers to maintain a conscious awareness of this power and how it may show up in the treatment room.

Malin Fors (2021) describes a number of power dynamics that infiltrate the therapeutic relationship, two of which are particularly relevant when it comes to working with kinky clients. "Professional power," Fors posits, involves the inherent imbalance that accompanies a professional therapeutic relationship: "The clinician has extensive information about the patient; the patient lacks similar data about the clinician. The therapist is paid to see the patient, keeps a medical record, and in most cases, has more extensive psychological knowledge"

DOI: 10.4324/9781003312833-10

(Fors, 2021). It is no secret that this type of asymmetry will exist within a therapeutic relationship. Due to the sensitive nature of clinical work, maintaining healthy boundaries is crucial and some of this involves sitting responsibly in this position of power. Fors also refers to this kind of power as overt, as it can be explicitly seen in cases that include "reporting to child services, involuntary hospitalization, assigning a diagnosis, and so on" (ibid). Whether or not clinicians want power to show up in the therapeutic space, it is unavoidable in these types of situations. When BDSM dynamics are presented in a clinical setting, it is even more vital to remain mindful of how this power manifests. Therapists must consciously ensure that they are not irresponsibly leaning into professional power, which often looks like clinicians projecting assumptions about BDSM dynamics rather than allowing clients to lead as the experts in their own lives.

Another form of power discussed by Fors is "socio-political power," which encompasses "various issues of external social power as they enter the therapeutic space" (Fors, 2021). While throughout a therapist's educational journey, immense attention is given to understanding theoretical orientations, diagnoses, legal and ethical issues, and more, it remains necessary to understand the ways in which social privilege shows up in the therapeutic space. Black and Stone define "social privilege" as:

> any entitlement, sanction, power, immunity, and advantage or right granted or conferred by the dominant group to a person or group solely by birth-right membership in prescribed identities. Social privilege is expressed through some combination of the following domains: race/ethnicity, gender, sexual orientation, SES, age, differing degrees of ableness, and religious affiliation.
>
> Black & Stone, 2005

Social privilege is interwoven into all relational dynamics. It is imperative for clinicians to be aware of how it shows up in the clinical setting, as it can undoubtedly impact the therapeutic relationship if not carefully considered. Professional power and socio-political power can also intertwine, further impacting the therapeutic relationship.

> Therapeutic relationships consist, at a minimum, of a highly educated trained professional with knowledge of therapy, interfacing with clients from varying backgrounds who are seeking help. From the beginning, this establishes a structural hierarchy in the therapy process, with the therapist being in a position of greater privilege. However, other aspects of intersectionality affect the therapeutic relationship as well, stemming

from differences in therapist and client social locations. For example, a white therapist is "doubly empowered" by race and professional position with clients of color, while a therapist of color is empowered by only the therapist position (Watts-Jones, 2010, p. 409). In instances where the therapist possesses multiple dimensions of marginalized identities (such as a female therapist of color), working with a client from a more dominant social position (such as a white male) may lead to the dynamic feeling "flipped" in the room, where the client is perceived to hold greater power despite the therapist's professional position. Regardless of who holds greater social privilege in the therapeutic relationship, finding a way to address, when appropriate, dynamics of power and privilege differences can be crucial to establishing a positive therapeutic alliance.

Pettyjohn et al., 2020

While conversations around privilege are beginning to integrate into many more clinical settings, we must continue to turn toward them rather than away from them. Approaching clients without addressing and deeply understanding how each clinician's social privilege is inherently present may severely impact the therapeutic relationship. Including privilege as a central area of focus in educational curricula is necessary, especially when clinicians will be working with erotically marginalized populations.

We view any attempt to train culturally competent counselors without a focus on privilege as inappropriate and intentionally reinforcing the oppression of the status quo. Furthermore, failure to address the dynamics of privilege and oppression within the counseling profession and the counseling relationship is likely to produce counselors with restricted emotional, intellectual, and psychological development, thus lowering the overall effectiveness of the counseling profession.

Black & Stone, 2005

The importance of recognizing personal privilege is not exclusive to the mental health field; it is vital within all professions, particularly when folks are engaging with kink-identified individuals. As noted many times throughout this book, kinksters are not *only* kinksters; they are kinky people with a variety of intersecting identities that all play a role in their life experiences. Whether in a medical, legal, educational, or clinical setting, an emphasis on understanding, addressing, and further adjusting is crucial when working with this population. Social power and privilege and how they can influence care must be consistently and intentionally addressed.

There are several ways to work toward a more inclusive and affirming practice, many of which require significant internal work. Expanding on the works of Pettyjohn et al. (2020), Salmon (2017), Brown and Lengyell (2022), and Goerlich (2020), the following is a list of personal actions that can start building a framework for an affirming practice:

- Recognize the dimensions of identity that differ between yourself and the person in your care.
- Reflect on the ways in which you may unintentionally oppress or reinforce problematic power dynamics within the professional relationship.
- Acknowledge the contextual factors going on in society at large and how they may be impacting the individual.
- Recognize the value of the individual's lived experience; regardless of your educational, personal, or professional experience, your client is the primary expert in their life.
- Invest in ongoing educational discussion and prioritize seeking critical knowledge, particularly regarding identities that are unfamiliar to you.
- Participate in ongoing self-reflection: sit in discomfort, embrace humility, and seek consultation should you find yourself approaching kinky individuals with judgment.

For folks who have not yet considered their own privilege and how it may be impacting the lives of those they engage with, this work will feel extremely challenging. This is normal and, frankly, necessary. Sitting in discomfort is part of this work and a commitment to engaging in self-reflection can mean the difference between helping or harming our clients.

THE KINK-AFFIRMING PROVIDER

When working with an erotically marginalized community, such as the kink community, it is critical to ensure that clinicians are providing competent care. It is both a professional and ethical responsibility of all clinicians to assess their gaps in kink knowledge and work diligently toward filling them. This is particularly important as research suggests a high likelihood of clinicians will see at least one kinky client throughout their careers (Helfer, 2022; Kelsey, 2012). Further, given the lack of competency that many clinicians feel when working with this population and the lack of educational opportunities to gain kink-related knowledge during graduate school, clinicians must take it upon themselves to undertake the necessary education to work with kinksters. If not, while they may be kink aware, they may not necessarily be kink-affirming. So, what does it mean to be "kink-affirming"? My co-author, Stefani Goerlich, described it beautifully in an interview with Lawrence Rubin:

> Kink-affirming practice is the understanding that kink is not just something that we need to know about. Kink-affirming practice understands that kink is its own distinct subculture, with strengths and resources and things that we can use in clinical work with our clients, and that we can leverage their kink identities in our treatment planning, in our intervention strategies, and really work with that in the same way that we would use any other aspect of our clients' identities. So it's taking it beyond "I understand this" and moving it into "This is a key part of your identity. And we are going to weave this into our work.
>
> Rubin, 2021

As Dr. Goerlich notes, a thorough level of education and experience is necessary to become a kink-affirming provider. While this may seem daunting (if you have read this far, you are already doing a great job!), many resources can provide guidance on this educational journey. However, without the proper foundation, it can be challenging to continue building toward becoming a kink-affirming clinician. Thus, mental health professionals can begin by approaching counseling from a sex-affirming framework:

> A sex-affirming framework of counseling centers on the assertion that sex is a natural part of the human experience and offers important contributions to clients' mental and emotional wellbeing, relational health, and overall life satisfaction. Counselors can exemplify a sex-affirming stance with clients by normalizing the topic of sexual discussion with congruence and comfort. Sexuality is also viewed as expansive, emergent, and pluralistic—that is, counselors acknowledge that sexuality is experienced in innumerable ways that are shaped by the client's unique social, cultural, and environmental contexts. Although values related to consent, equality, and responsibility are emphasized, sex-affirming counselors also recognize that there is no one "right" kind of sexuality and that all individuals create their own meanings related to sexual morality. In other words, sex-affirming counselors regard all sexual behaviors occurring between informed and consenting partners as potentially healthy and beneficial forms of intimacy.
>
> A sex-affirming approach to counseling is also responsive to multicultural diversity and intersectionality. Clients that possess marginalized identities (e.g., LGBTQ+ individuals, people of Color, people with

disabilities, people from impoverished backgrounds) often face increased sexual health risks, such as decreased access to sexual healthcare and increased sexual stigmatization (World Health Organization, 2011). As such, counselors must recognize how discrimination systems such as white supremacy, patriarchy, and cisheteronormativity inform societal values about sexuality, as well as how discriminatory sexual norms may impact clients' sexual wellness. As each client possesses multiple identities that contribute to their unique position of privilege and oppression, counselors should explore the sexual health implications of their clients' intersectional lived experiences.

Litam & Speciale, 2021

As clinicians become familiar with a sex-affirming way of approaching client work, they can begin building upon that framework to work toward becoming a kink-affirming provider. An excellent place to start when building toward gaining competency in working with kinky clients is the Kink Clinical Guidelines. "Over a two-year period, a team of 20 experienced clinicians and researchers created these clinical practice guidelines for working with people involved with kink, incorporating an extensive literature review and documentation of clinical expertise." (Sprott et al., 2023) The Kink Clinical Guidelines provide a framework for working with kinky people and can be utilized to highlight gaps in knowledge. The guidelines are as follows:

- **Guideline 1:** Clinicians understand that "kink" is used as an umbrella term for a wide range of consensual erotic or intimate behaviors, fantasies, relationships, and identities.
- **Guideline 2:** Clinicians will be aware of their professional competence and scope of practice when working with clients who are exploring kink or who are kink-identified, and will consult, obtain supervision, and/or refer as appropriate to best serve their clients.
- **Guideline 3:** Clinicians understand that kink fantasies, interests, behaviors, relationships, and/or identities, by themselves, do not indicate the presence of psychopathology, a mental disorder, or the inability of individuals to control their behavior.
- **Guideline 4:** Clinicians understand that kink is not necessarily a response to trauma, including abuse.
- **Guideline 5:** Clinicians recognize that kink intersects with other identities in ways that may shape how kink is expressed and experienced.

- **Guideline 6:** Clinicians understand that kink may sometimes facilitate the exploration and expression of a range of gender, relationship, and sexuality interests and identities.
- **Guideline 7:** Clinicians recognize how stigma, discrimination, and violence directed at people involved in kink can affect their health and wellbeing.
- **Guideline 8:** Clinicians understand the centrality of consent and how it is managed in kink interactions and power-exchange relationships.
- **Guideline 9:** Clinicians understand that kink experiences can lead to healing, personal growth, and empowerment.
- **Guideline 10:** Clinicians consider how generational differences can influence kink behaviors and identities.
- **Guideline 11:** Clinicians understand that kink interests may be recognized at any age.
- **Guideline 12:** Clinicians understand that there is a wide variety of family structures among kink-identified individuals.
- **Guideline 13:** Clinicians do not assume that kink involvement has a negative effect on parenting.
- **Guideline 14:** Clinicians do not assume that any concern arising in therapy is caused by kink.
- **Guideline 15:** Clinicians understand that reparative or conversion therapies are unethical. Similarly, clinicians avoid attempts to eradicate consensual kink behaviors and identities.
- **Guideline 16:** Clinicians understand that distress about kink may reflect internalized stigma, oppression, and negativity rather than evidence of a disorder.
- **Guideline 17:** Clinicians should evaluate their own biases, values, attitudes, and feelings about kink and address how those can affect their interactions with clients on an ongoing basis.
- **Guideline 18:** Clinicians understand that societal stereotypes about kink may affect the client's presentation in treatment and the process of therapy.
- **Guideline 19:** Clinicians understand that intimate partner violence/domestic violence (IPV/DV) can co-exist with kink activities or relationships. Clinicians should ensure their assessments for intimate partner violence/domestic violence are kink informed.
- **Guideline 20:** Clinicians strive to remain informed about the current scientific literature about kink and avoid misuse or misrepresentation of findings and methods.

Scan to view in-depth descriptions of each of the Kink Clinical Guidelines.

Figure 10.1 Kink Clinical Guidelines (QR code)

- **Guideline 21:** Clinicians support the development of professional education and training on kink-related issues.
- **Guideline 22:** Clinicians make reasonable efforts to familiarize themselves with health, educational, and community resources relevant to clients who are exploring kink or who have a kink identity.
- **Guideline 23:** Clinicians support social change to reduce stigma regarding kink.

While this list is specifically geared toward mental health clinicians, it can be helpful for a variety of careers where someone may be interacting with or working with a kinky person. Adherence to these guidelines is indeed an excellent step; however, as overwhelming as it might seem, it is not the only one. Becoming a kink-affirming provider takes time, energy, and intention. Just as the world is ever-changing, so too are the many subcultures within the kink community. A deep understanding of the kink community is not simply achieved by reading one book or attending one class; it is achieved by a commitment to pursuing ongoing education and learning not only from kink experts but, more importantly, from those with lived experience. At the end of the day, no one knows kinksters better than kinksters.

EFFECTIVE INTERVENTIONS

We know that the majority of kinky clients do not seek therapy *because* they are kinky; they are simply kinky people in need of support as they work through general mental health or life-stage concerns. However there will be times when our clients seek treatment because they feel shame or guilt around their desires. In some rare instances, we may also encounter clients who are engaging in problematic behaviors that put them at legitimate risk of harm—either judicially, physically, or relationally. When these clients seek treatment, they can and should be treated in the same way we address any of our kinky clients: with affirmation, acceptance, and unconditional positive regard for their humanity and their desires, even as we explore potential behavioral changes that may be needed for optimal health and wellbeing. We can do this by centering interventions grounded in the ideals of intimate justice and pleasure equity in our work with all clients—kinky or vanilla. These interventions, first published in Stefani's early book, *Kink-Affirming Practice: Culturally Competent Therapy from The Leather Chair,* include the following:

- **Decouple** BDSM/kink and intercourse in your mind: don't assume that your kinky client is sexually active or that sex is a priority for them (Berry & Lezos, 2017).
- **Ask** your client to describe what they want when it comes to sex and relationships. Ask them if they believe they are entitled to have these things in their life (McClelland, 2014).
- **Express** curiosity about the somatic aspects of your client's sexuality: their body image, the way in which size (larger or smaller) impacts their play, and any experiences of disability or pain (Kauffman et al., 2007).
- **De-center** penetrative sex and orgasm as indicators of sexual success and encourage clients to define satisfying sexuality for themselves (McClelland, 2012).
- **Introduce** discussions of gender roles and messages about what it means to be a "real ___." Encourage clients to process how they have internalized these messages in relation to their kink identity (Pittagora, 2015).
- **Discuss** the messages that your clients receive from partners, religious leaders, other healthcare providers, pop culture and the media, etc. about their sexual identity and desires (Sand, 2019).
- **Avoid** diagnostic attribution errors, such as assuming that a client's desires are rooted in trauma, that their relationship structure is intrinsically maladaptive, or that their BDSM desires are symptoms of a mental health concern (Sloan, 2019).
- **Recognize** the importance of equality of expectation within power exchange and affirm that your client's relationship dynamic can be both unequal and still equitable (Goerlich, 2020).

- **Challenge** internalized shame and inadequacy within your client and help them to move toward a mindset of deservingness (Allendar & Longman, 2014).
- **Be willing** to name systemic and institutional oppression experienced by your client. Ask how, if at all, their experiences of oppression impact their kink identity and/or BDSM play (Constantinides et al., 2019).
- **Embrace** flexibility and ambiguity and empower your client to experiment with identities and roles in order to find their own most authentic self. Recognize that this can, and likely will, evolve over time (Berry & Lezos, 2017).
- **Make** pleasure a theme within your clinical work. Help your client identify barriers to pleasure and identify ways to overcome or mitigate these barriers (Baggett et al., 2017).

BEST PRACTICES

Within the domain of mental health professions—including disciplines such as marriage and family therapy, clinical counseling, and social work—ethical guidelines inform how we engage with and approach our clients. These guidelines are particularly salient for providers working with members of marginalized communities and play a pivotal role in shaping our interactions with clients. The established frameworks for upholding ethical standards provide an excellent foundation for clinical practice and ensure that our clients are receiving the best possible care. However, cultivating a space that is inclusive, affirming, and sex-positive takes more than simply abiding by a list of guidelines. As professionals, we must go beyond the standards and create a new way of engaging that includes identities that have been overlooked or excluded. Not only must we look at the individual experiences of our kinky clients; we must expand our knowledge to encompass the many systems that impact those clients. A critical part of our work is helping clients navigate systems that work to omit and erase their identities and, importantly, learn how to mitigate risk when engaging with those systems.

KINK AND THE LAW

As discussed at various points in this book, consent is critical when engaging with BDSM; and while consent is certainly a pillar of kink activity and vital for healthy kink engagement, there are circumstances where consent violations have been reported. In an online survey of nearly 3,000 kinky participants, the NCSF found that 25.5% of respondents reported a consent violation; and that of those violations, only 3.5% were reported to police (Bowling et al., 2022). While it is no surprise that the legal system has failed sexual assault survivors time and time again, there are sexual rights advocacy groups and activists that are working to fix our very broken system.

The kink community is known to be self-regulating; but while this may be helpful for those in the community who are seeking emotional support, it does not help when the law becomes involved. As a provider working with kinky individuals—whether in a legal, medical, educational, or clinical context—it is important to understand consent both as an ethical principle and as a legal principle.

- **Consent as an ethical principle:** "BDSM activities are based on the ethical principle that what we do—whether it is a specific scene or a relationship—is done by informed agreement amongst all of the participants. Our ethics require that all the participants communicate what they agree to do and not to do, as well as the nature of the relationship that they agree to enter. Each participant has a responsibility to reach as complete an understanding as possible of the desires and limits of the other participants. In short, consent as an ethical concept is one of mutual and informed consent (National Coalition for Sexual Freedom, 2021).
- **Consent as a legal principle:** "The legal issue of consent is more narrow and specific. It relates only to a specific activity or scene and only to the question of whether the person receiving the BDSM stimulation agreed in advance to do that act. The legal issue arises when someone is harmed or injured by a BDSM act, and the person who committed that act denies criminal liability on the ground that the other person gave prior consent to the act in question. The extent to which such consent—even if clearly given—is a defense to criminal prosecution has been greatly limited by U.S. courts (ibid).

With the intent of empowering sexual assault survivors and destigmatizing consensual BDSM engagement, the NCSF, along with various additional professional organizations, has worked for over a decade to pursue a change regarding consent laws. One of their primary guiding intentions is highlighting the conflation of crime and consensual BDSM. When the law states that causing physical harm—whether injury or intense pain—to another individual is a criminal offense, it disregards the ways in which BDSM participants engage with one another. Thus, while in many cases physical harm is indeed a criminal act, by this rigid definition, simply engaging in BDSM can be defined as criminal.

> The definitions of assault, abuse and other such crimes involving infliction of physical harm, as well as the provisions (if any) dealing with consent as a defense to such criminal charges, are matters of individual states' laws. There is no federal law in this area. The laws vary from state to state, and many state laws on assault do not mention consent as a defense. There are, however, a number of state assault statutes that do provide for consent as a defense. Such statutes invariably place limits on the consent defense, both in terms of the degree of harm and in terms of the way in which consent is given and the types of people who cannot legally give their consent.
>
> National Coalition for Sexual Freedom, 2021

In 2021, the American Law Institute approved the revised Model Penal Code on Sexual Assault, including an updated definition of "consent" for sexual activity, which is particularly important as "over 20 states have no definition of consent in their sexual assault law, and there is no uniform legal definition of consent" (National Coalition for Sexual Freedom, 2021). These ground-breaking changes, if adopted into state law, would "decriminalize BDSM activities in connection with sexual penetration, oral sex or sexual contact" (National Coalition for Sexual Freedom, 2019). The updated definitions are listed below:

New Definition of Consent to Sex

(a) "Consent" for purposes of Article 213 means a person's willingness to engage in a specific act of sexual penetration or sexual contact.

(b) Consent may be express or it may be inferred from behavior—both action and inaction—in the context of all the circumstances.

(c) Neither verbal nor physical resistance is required to establish that consent is lacking, but their absence may be considered, in the context of all the circumstances, in determining whether there was consent.

(d) Notwithstanding subsection (3)(b) of this Section, consent is ineffective when it occurs in circumstances described in Sections [reserved].

(e) Consent may be revoked or withdrawn any time before or during the act of sexual penetration or sexual contact. A clear verbal refusal—such as "No," "Stop," or "Don't"—establishes the lack of consent or the revocation or withdrawal of previous consent. Lack of consent or revocation or withdrawal of consent may be overridden by subsequent consent.

American Law Institute, 2016

New Definition of Consent to BDSM

Affirmative Defense of Explicit Prior Permission

You may personally give another person explicit prior permission to use or threaten to use physical force or restraint or to inflict or threaten to inflict any harm in connection with an act of sexual penetration, oral sex, or sexual contact, as long as it does not cause serious injury.

Permission is "explicit" when it is given orally or by written agreement:

(a) specifying that the actor may ignore the other party's expressions of unwillingness or other absence of consent;
(b) identifying the specific forms and extent of force, restraint, or threats that are permitted; and
(c) stipulating the specific words or gestures that will withdraw the permission.

American Law Institute, 2022

These updated definitions can help providers—and kinky folks—gain a better understanding of how consent is understood in a legal context. They further make clear the steps that must be taken to ensure that consent has been obtained. The NCSF has listed the following questions to obtain "explicit prior permission" for consent to kink activity. These questions are fundamental for all individuals who participate in kink:

- Did you agree to the specific acts you're going to do together, including if there's going to be any sexual contact like touching the breasts or genitals?
- Is everyone an adult and able to consent; they're not under the influence, in subspace, having a mental health crisis, or a significant reduction in capacity?
- Did you discuss the risks and agree as to how intense it will be? Note: You can't seriously injure someone, even if they consented to the act.
- Do you have a way to stop at any time-even if you're doing consensual non-consent-like a safe word or safe signal?
- What verbal or physical resistance did you agree that it's okay to ignore, ie. in roleplay or power exchange?

National Coalition for Sexual Freedom, 2021

CREATING AN AFFIRMING SPACE

> The foremost important strategy in working with this population is the counselor's ability to critically self-examine personal beliefs about BDSM and consider the ways in which these beliefs may impact the therapeutic relationship.
>
> —Litam & Speciale, 2021

Given the highly stigmatized nature of kink participation, it is unsurprising that many kinky folks choose to keep their kink identities a secret. Various studies indicate that kink disclosure may be prohibited because of a fear of how providers will respond. One 2006 study involving 175 participants revealed that more than one-quarter refrained from disclosing their participation in kink activities. Reasons cited included the perception that it was unrelated to their therapy objectives or fear of potential negative reactions from therapists (Kolmes et al., 2006). Similarly, a study of 115 BDSM practitioners indicated that fewer than half had divulged their kink identity to healthcare providers, primarily due to concerns about facing stigma (Waldura et al., 2016). Beyond the fear of stigma, individuals within the kink community express anxieties regarding the pathologization of their practices and identities; and therapists erroneously associating kink activities with self-harm or abuse (Nevard, 2019).

What is particularly jarring about this information is the implications for disclosure of kink identity in mental and physical healthcare spaces—particularly when services could be beneficial (e.g., processing and understanding newly discovered parts of one's identity) or even necessary (e.g., if an injury occurs during a scene). It is crucial to consciously assess barriers that may hinder or prevent the disclosure of one's kink identity, particularly given the importance of the therapeutic alliance in effective psychotherapy (Graham, 2014). Kink research continues to reveal that disclosure can be a problem for kinky folks, so it is vital that clinicians create a space conducive to open and honest dialog.

Not only do kinky folks hold fear that they may have negative experiences with mental healthcare providers; many of them have already had those experiences, deterring them further from kink identity disclosure. When assessing negative therapeutic interactions, Kolmes, Stock, and Moser (2006) reported several experiences of "biased, inadequate, or inappropriate care to a BDSM client in psychotherapy." These experiences included:

1) Therapists considering BDSM to be unhealthy,
2) Requiring a client to give up BDSM activities in order to continue in treatment,
3) Confusing BDSM with abuse,
4) Having to educate the therapist about BDSM,
5) Assuming that BDSM interests are indicative of past family/spousal abuse, and
6) Therapists misrepresenting their expertise by stating that they are BDSM-positive when they are not actually knowledgeable about BDSM practice

Kolmes et al., 2006

These types of interactions highlight the importance of kink education and how therapists' bias can create an environment that is truly harmful to clients. Thus, to create a space for disclosure, clinicians must actively work toward creating a more affirming space. Aside from learning from the ways in which kinky folks have experienced positive interactions related to BDSM—including "therapist(s) being open to reading/learning more about BDSM, therapist(s) showing comfort in talking about BDSM issues, and therapists who understand and promote [consent frameworks]" (ibid)—therapists can further indicate their openness even before a kinky client walks through their physical or virtual door.

The following are additional ways to create affirming spaces beyond the internal and educational work:

- Ensure that your website, bios, and promotional materials indicate that you work with kink/BDSM.
- Within the therapy space (whether in an office or virtual), try to have books, symbols, or decor in sight that may indicate it is a safe space (similar to LGTBQIA+ clinicians having Pride flags visible).
- If kink/BDSM is your specialty, be mindful that paperwork does not assume "normative" relational structures and types. For example, instead of "single/married/divorced/other," you may include a more open-ended question, such as "Please describe your current relational dynamics (single, partnered/monogamous, partnered/non-monogamous, etc.)"

- Network openly as a kink-affirming provider. Ensure that any referrals that come your way have already become aware of the type of work that you do.
- Attend conferences, conventions, and other events that cater to the communities you work with. It is extremely important to remain mindful and respectful of community etiquette, especially if you are not a part of the community that you serve. Pay attention to spaces that are meant only for community members.
- Should you have the means, time, and ability to advocate for the communities that you are serving, volunteer your time, join activist groups, and work on the macro level toward a better future for your clients.

It takes time and effort to create a space that is conducive to openness around kink identity. However, identity disclosure will always come down to the client's readiness and should never be pushed or forced. All we can do is open the door to the conversation and allow our clients to make the decision about whether they would like to come in.

ADDITIONAL RESOURCES

Unequal By Design: Counseling Power Dynamic Relationships by Sabrina Popp and Raven Kaldera

The Leather Couch: Clinical Practice with Kinky Clients and *Kink-Affirming Practice: Culturally Competent Therapy from The Leather Chair* by Stefani Goerlich

The Queer Mental Health Workbook by Brendan J. Dunlap

Integrating Geek Culture into Therapeutic Practice: The Clinician's Guide to Geek Therapy by Anthony M. Bean, Emory S. Daniel Jr., and Sarah A. Hays (eds.)

Relationally Queer by Silva Neves and Dominic Davies (eds.)

Erotically Queer by Silva Neves and Dominic Davies (eds.)

CONCLUSION

This small book has covered quite a large amount of content. Any chapter or subsection could warrant an entire volume of its own, and—as our recommendations at the end of each chapter demonstrate—many of these titles are available for those who wish to take their learning deeper. We encourage you to use *BDSM & Kink: The Basics* as a starting point on your path toward greater cultural competency, enhanced clinical skill, and kink-affirming practice. Our thoughts should not be considered definitive: the BDSM/kink community is incredibly diverse, encompasses multiple subcultures, includes people from all backgrounds, and is incorporated into many different types of relationships. No single text could ever speak to the full breadth of the BDSM/kink experience. Likewise, no single etiological theory, diagnostic code, or treatment modality can apply to every kinkster you'll work with—even those who use the same identifiers, form the same relationship agreements, or engage in the same erotic behaviors. We encourage you to keep learning and, specifically, engaging with content created by the BDSM/kink community.

The impact of minority stress, social isolation, and kink stigma cannot be understated, and clinical practitioners are well positioned to mitigate these harms. The way in which each clinician connects with their clients, builds rapport, assesses risk and safety, and engages in the mutual work of therapy can either alleviate these experiences or reinforce them. We hope this book has offered a variety of insights, tools, and suggestions that you can put into practice immediately. As you do, the authors would like to leave you with a final recommendation:

The paraphilias should ALWAYS be a diagnosis of exclusion.

Throughout these pages, we have explored the history and evolution of sexual dysfunctions and explained the calculus of Time + Place that has been used for centuries to determine who is deemed socially acceptable and who is deemed deviant. While historically misunderstood and pathologized, BDSM is an ever-evolving, deeply connecting, and expansive way of relating. Looking into the community allows us to see immense connection, intimacy, community, playfulness, and pleasure. As we write this conclusion, we are in the early days of 2024 and the social dialog around "deviance" versus "the mainstream" has only intensified. Trans rights are under attack. LGBTQIA+ people and sexuality educators are labeled "groomers." And those of us who engage in the work of clinical sexology and relationship therapies are being asked to define who should be trusted and who should be treated.

Each of us has the capacity to speak from a position of clinical ethics, scientific research, and the wisdom of our clients' lived experience. We can choose—through our diagnostics and through our dialogs—either to speak up for our marginalized clients or to perpetuate the historical harms that our field has so often inflicted upon those who are different. We have an ethical obligation to explore every other differential diagnosis before applying a stigmatizing label to our clients; and the risk of pathologization to which we expose our clients when we use these diagnostic codes should lead us to be highly judicious in when and how we make these diagnoses. We hope this book has given practitioners the context and insights necessary to enhance their diagnostic skills. Further, we hope that our readers have been able to open their hearts and minds to understanding and embracing the varied ways in which people connect with one another—and that you will continue on this journey with us toward a more sex-positive, inclusive future.

BIBLIOGRAPHY

Abel, G. G., Coffey, L., & Osborn, C. A. (2008). Sexual arousal patterns: Normal and deviant. *Psychiatric Clinics of North America, 31*(4), 643–655.

Abel, G. G. & Osborn, C. (1992). The paraphilias: The extent and nature of sexually deviant and criminal behavior. *Psychiatric Clinics of North America, 15*, 675–687.

Afana, E. D. (2021, August). Perception Correction: Addressing Social Stigmatization Around BDSM and Mental Health. https://scholarworks.sjsu. edu/cgi/viewcontent.cgi?article=8741&context=etd_theses

ALDF. (2010, December 15). Case Study: Animal Fighting—Michael Vick. https://aldf.org/case/case-study-animal-fighting-michael-vick/

Alegre, S. M. (2018). Sex and the humaniform robot: Between science fiction and robosexuality. *Robotics Meets the Humanities*. Barcelona, Spain: International Conference on Intelligent Robots.
https://ddd.uab.cat/pub/poncom/2018/200599/SMARTIN_Sex_and_the_ Humaniform_Robot.pdf).

Allendar, D. B. & Longman, III, T. (2014). *God Loves Sex: An Honest Conversation About Sexual Desire and Holiness*. Grand Rapids, MI: Baker Books.

Ambler, J. K., Lee, E. M., Klement, K. R., Loewald, T., Comber, E. M., Hanson, S. A., & Sagarin, B. J. (2017). Consensual BDSM facilitates role-specific altered states of consciousness: A preliminary study. *Psychology of Consciousness: Theory, Research and Practice, 4*(1), 75–91. https://doi.org/10.1037/cns0000097.

American Law Institute (2016). Updated "Consent" Definition. https://www.ali. org/news/articles/updated-consent-definition/

American Law Institute (2022). Model Penal Code: Sexual Assault and Related Offenses. https://www.ali.org/media/filer_public/05/8e/058eb1a1-5c05-40d5-83db-407445e510b2/sexual_assault_-_td6.pdf

Ansara, Y. G. (2019). Trauma psychotherapy with people involved in BDSM/kink: Five common misconceptions and five essential clinical skills. *Psychotherapy and Counselling Journal of Australia, 7*(2).

APA. (2013). *The Diagnostic and Statistical Manual of Mental Disorders, 5th Edition.* Washington D.C.: American Psychiatric Association.

APA Dictionary. (n.d.). Definition of Bestiality. American Psychological Association. https://dictionary.apa.org/bestiality

APA Dictionary. (n.d.). Definition of Zoophilia. American Psychological Association. https://dictionary.apa.org/zoophilia

Artsy Editorial. (2013, September 24). What is Shunga? *Artsy.* https://www.artsy.net/article/editorial-what-is-shunga

Australian Associated Press. (2018, June 20). Sex assault charges dropped against fetish website user 'The Wolf'. *Sydney Morning Herald.* https://www.smh.com.au/national/nsw/sex-assault-charges-dropped-against-fetish-website-user-the-wolf-20180620-p4zmpl.html

Baggett, R.L., Eisen, E., Gonzales-Rivas, S., Olson, L.A., Cameron, R.P., & Mona, L. (2017). Sex-positive assessment and treatment among female trauma survivors. *Journal of Clinical Psychology 73*(8), 965–974.

Barber, T. (2004). Deviation as a key to innovation: Understanding a culture of the future. *Foresight, 6*(3), 141–153. doi10.1108/14636680410547744.

Bastian, B., Jetten, J., Hornsey, M. J., & Leknes, S. (2014). The positive consequences of pain: A biopsychosocial approach. *Personality and Social Psychology Review, 18*(3), 256–279. https://doi.org/10.1177/1088868314527831.

Bauer, R. (2010). Non-monogamy in queer BDSM communities: Putting the sex back into alternative relationship practices and discourse. In M. Barker & D. Langdridge (eds.), *Understanding Non-monogamies* (pp. 154–165). New York, NY: Routledge.

Bauer, R. (2018). Bois and grrrls meet their daddies and mommies on gender playgrounds: Gendered age play in the les-bi-trans-queer BDSM communities. *Sexualities, 21*(1–2), 139–155.

Baumeister, R. F. (1998). Masochism as escape from self. *The Journal of Sex Research, (25)*1, 28–59.

Bedbible Research Center. (2023, September 29). Most Common Fetishes. https://bedbible.com/what-is-the-most-common-fetish-statistics/

Beech, A. R. & Harkins, L. (2012). DSM-IV paraphilia: Descriptions, demographics and treatment interventions. *Aggression and Violent Behavior, 17*(6), 527–539. https://doi.org/10.1016/j.avb.2012.07.008

Beech A. R., Miner M. H., & Thornton D. (2016). Paraphilias in the DSM-5. *Annual Review of Clinical Psychology, 12,* 383–406. doi: 10.1146/annurev-clinpsy-021815-093330. PMID: 26772210.

Bentham, J. (1780). *An Introduction to the Principles of Morals and Legislation.* London, UK: Oxford.

Berger, P., Berner, W., Boltrerauer, J., Guitierrez, K., & Berger, K. (1999). Sadistic personality disorder in sex offenders: Relationship to antisocial personality disorder and sexual sadism. *Journal of Personality Disorders, 13*(2), 175–186. doi 10.1521/pedi.1999.13.2.175.

Berry, M. D. & Lezos, A. M. (2017). Inclusive sex therapy practices: A qualitative study of the techniques sex therapists use when working with diverse populations. *Sexual and Relationship Therapy, 32*(1), 2–21.

Bhadelia, A., De Lima, L., Arreola-Ornelas, H., Kwete, X. J., Rodiguez, N. M., & Knaul, F. M. (2019). Solving the global crisis in access to pain relief: Lessons from country actions. *American Journal of Public Health, 109*(1), 58–60.

Bhatia K, Parekh U. Frotteurism. [Updated 2023 Aug 8]. In: StatPearls [Internet]. Treasure Island (FL): StatPearls Publishing; 2024 Jan-. Available from: https://www.ncbi.nlm.nih.gov/books/NBK563260/

Black, L. L. & Stone, D. (2005). Expanding the definition of privilege: The concept of social privilege. *Journal of Multicultural Counseling and Development, 33*(4), 243–255. https://doi.org/10.1002/j.2161-1912.2005.tb00020.x

Borzarth, J. D. (2024, January 8). The Core Values of the Person-Centered Approach. Association for the Development of the Person-Centered Approach. https://adpca.org/the-core-values-of-the-person-centered-approach/

Bowman, C. P. (2014). Women's masturbation: Experiences of sexual empowerment in a primarily sex-positive sample. *Psychology of Women Quarterly, 38*(3), 363–378. https://doi.org/10.1177/0361684313514855

Breithaupt, F. (2018). The bad things we do because of empathy. *Interdisciplinary Science Reviews, 43*(2), 166–174.

Breithaupt, F. (2019). *The Dark Sides of Empathy.* Ithaca, NY/London, UK: Cornell University Press.

Brennan, F., Carr, D. B., & Cousins, M. (2007). Pain management: A fundamental human right. *Pain Medicine, 105*(1), 205–221.

Brown A., Barker E. D., & Rahman Q. (2020). A systematic scoping review of the prevalence, etiological, psychological, and interpersonal factors associated with BDSM. *Journal of Sex Research, 57*(6), 781–811. doi: 10.1080/00224499.2019.1665619. PMID: 31617765.

Brown, B. (2012). *Daring Greatly: How the Courage to be Vulnerable Transforms the Way We Live, Love, Parent and Lead.* New York, NY: Penguin.

Brown, J. & Lengyel, M. (2022). Psychotherapists' efforts to increase awareness of social privilege. *Counseling and Psychotherapy Research, 23*(1), 84–95. 10.1002/capr.12539.

Buaban, J. (2021). On masturbation: Religious purity and institutional hegemony in Abrahamic religions and Buddhism. *Prajñā Vihāra: Journal of Philosophy and Religion, 22*(1), 55.

Buckels, E. E. (2018). *The Psychology of Everyday Sadism.* Vancouver, BC: The University of British Columbia.

Buckels, E. E., Jones, D. N., & Paulhus, D. L. (2013). Behavioral confirmation of everyday sadism. *Psychological Science, 24*(11), 1–9, http://pss.sagepub.com/content/early/2013/09/09/0956797613490749.

Bullough, V. (2003). Masturbation: A historical overview. *Journal of Psychology Human Sexuality, 14*(2–3), 17–33. doi: 10.1300/J056v14n02_03

Camacho, N. A. (2023, May 25). National Masturbation Month: A surgeon general's firing inspired the celebration. *Teen Vogue.* https://www.teenvogue.com/story/national-masturbation-month-history

Carlström, C. (2018). BDSM, becoming and the flows of desire. *Culture, Health & Sexuality, 24*(4), 404–415. doi: 10.1080/13691058.2018.1485969

Carvalheira, A & Leal, I. (2012). Masturbation among women: Associated factors and sexual response in a Portuguese community sample. *Journal of Sex & Marital Therapy, 39*(4). 10.1080/0092623X.2011.628440.

Cascalheira, C., Thomson, A., & Wignall, L. (2021). "A certain evolution": A phenomenological study of 24/7 BDSM and negotiating consent. *Psychology & Sexuality, 13*(2). 10.1080/19419899.2021.1901771.

Charleston, L. (2019, July 20). The brutal anti-masturbation devices of the Victorian era. *New Zealand Herald.* https://www.nzherald.co.nz/life-style/the-brutal-anti-masturbation-devices-of-the-victorian-era/BA3ABBTE2RP3LBY7BOEKHYKVMI/

Cito, G., Micelli, E., Cocci, A., Polloni, G., Russo, G. I., Coccia, M. E., & Natali, A. (2021). The impact of the COVID-19 quarantine on sexual life in Italy. *Urology, 147,* 37–42.

Clark-Flory, T. (2012, June 3). A BDSM Blacklist. *Salon.* https://www.salon.com/2012/06/03/a_bdsm_blacklist/

Cleveland Clinic. (2022). Masturbation: Facts and benefits. https://my.clevelandclinic.org/health/articles/24332-masturbation

Coleman, E. (2002). Masturbation as a means of achieving sexual health. *Journal of Psychology & Human Sexuality, 14*(2/3), 5–16.

Community-Academic Consortium for Research on Alternative Sexualities. (2023). Our Mission. https://carasresearch.org/our-mission/

Connolly, P. (2006). Psychological functioning of bondage/domination/sado-masochism (BDSM) practitioners. *Journal of Psychology & Human Sexuality, 18*(1), 79–120.

Constantinides, D., Sennot, S., & Chandler, D. (2019). *Sex Therapy with Erotically Marginalized Clients: Nine Principles of Clinical Support.* New York, NY: Routledge.

Cornell Law School. (2020, July). Pain and Suffering. Legal Information Institute. https://www.law.cornell.edu/wex/pain_and_suffering

Cowart, L. (2021). *Hurts So Good: The Science & Culture of Pain on Purpose.* New York, NY: PublicAffairs.

Cox, D., Lee, B., & Popky, D. (2022, May 3) How Prevalent Is Pornography? Institute for Family Studies. https://ifstudies.org/blog/how-prevalent-is-pornography

Crimmins, J. E. (2024, January 3). Jeremy Bentham. In E. Zalta & U. Nodelman (eds.) *The Stanford Encyclopedia of Philosophy* (Fall 2023 Edition). https://plato.stanford.edu/archives/fall2023/entries/bentham/

Cruz, A. (2016). *The Color of Kink: Black Women, BDSM, and Pornography.* New York, NY: NYU Press.

Csillag, V. (2014). Ordinary sadism in the consulting room. *Psychoanalytic Dialogues, 24*(4), 467–482. https://doi.org/10.1080/10481885.2014.932217.

Cumberpatch, C. (2000). People, Things, and Archeological Knowledge: An Exploration of the Significance of Fetishism in Archeology. Archaeology Data Service. https://archaeologydataservice.ac.uk/archives/view/assemblage/html/5/cumberpa.html

Damm, C., Dentato, M. P., & Busch, N. (2017). Unraveling intersecting identities: Understanding the lives of people who practice BDSM. *Psychology and Sexuality, 9*(1), 1–17.

Dan & J. D. (2009). *Two Knotty Boys Back on the Ropes*. San Francisco, CA: Green Candy Press.

Dancer PL, Kleinplatz PJ, Moser C (2006) 24/7 SM slavery. *Journal of Homosexuality 50*(2/3): 81–101.

Davis-Stober, C. P., McCarty, K. N., & McCarthy, D. M. (2019). Decision making and alcohol: Health policy implications. *Policy Insights from the Behavioral and Brain Sciences, 6*(1), 64–71 doi: 10.1177/2372732218818587.

De Neef, N., Huys, W., Morrens, M., & Coppens, V. (2019). Bondage-discipline, dominance-submission and sadomasochism (BDSM) from an integrative biopsychosocial perspective: A systematic review. *Sexual Medicine, 7*(2), 129–144. doi:10.1016/j.esxm.2019.02.002.

Deri, J. (2015). *Love's Refraction: Jealousy and Compersion in Queer Women's Polyamorous Relationships*. Toronto: University of Toronto Press.

Diver, K. (2005, April 3). Archaeologist finds 'oldest porn statue'. *The Guardian*. https://www.theguardian.com/world/2005/apr/04/arts.germany

Drouin, M., Hernandez, E., Machette, A., Garcia, J. R., & Boyd, R. L. (2023). An exploration of marks/injuries related to BDSM sexual experiences. *Sexual Medicine, 11*(3), qfad020. https://doi.org/10.1093/sexmed/qfad020

Dunn, B. (2023, August 8). Tackling the trust gap. *Forbes*. https://www.forbes.com/sites/forbesnonprofitcouncil/2023/08/08/tackling-the-trust-gap/?sh=18d6196f47fe

Earl, J. E. & Lucky, J. L. (2018). *How to Train Your Little: A DD/LG Guidebook*. CreateSpace Publishing.

Easton, D. & Hardy, J. (2001). *The New Bottoming Book*. Emeryville, CA: Greenery Press.

Essa, E. L. & Murray, C. I. (1999). Sexual play: When should you be concerned? *Childhood Education, 75*(4), 231–234.

Erickson, J. M. & Sagarin, B. J. (2021). The prosocial sadist? A comparison of BDSM sadism and everyday sadism. *Personality and Individual Differences, 176*(1), https://doi.org/10.1016/j.paid.2021.110723.

Eusei, D. & Delcea, C. (2020). *Theoretical-Experimental Models in Sexual and Paraphilic Dysfunctions*. Bologna, Italy: Filodiritto.

Fahs, B. & Frank, E. (2014) Notes from the back room: Gender, power, and (in)visibility in women's experiences of masturbation. *Journal of Sexual Research, 51*(3), 241–252. doi: 10.1080/00224499.2012.745474. Epub 2013 Apr 30. PMID: 23631671.

Fedoroff, J. P. (2020). *The Paraphilias: Changing Suits in the Evolution of Sexual Interest Paradigms*. New York, NY: Oxford.

Felluga, D. F. (2011, Jan 31). Fetishism. *Introductory Guide to Critical Theory*. Perdue University. https://www.cla.purdue.edu/academic/english/theory/psychoanalysis/definitions/fetishism.html#:~:text=Freud%20came%20to%20realize%20in,its%20power%20over%20the%20individual.

First, M. B. (2014). DSM-5 and paraphilic disorders. *Journal of the American Academy for Psychiatry Law, 42*(2), 191–201.

Frankfurther, D. (2019). *Magic and the Forces of Materiality*. Boston, MA: Brill.

Frayn, D. (1990). Intersubjective processes in psychotherapy. *Canadian Journal of Psychiatry, 35*(5), 434–438. doi: 10.1177/070674379003500513.

Freund, K. (1990). Courtship Disorder. In: W. L. Marshall, D. R. Laws & H. E. Barbaree (eds.) *Handbook of Sexual Assault*. Applied Clinical Psychology. Boston, MA: Springer. https://doi.org/10.1007/978-1-4899-0915-2_12

Gatzia, D. E. & Arnaud, S. (2022, October 17). Loving objects: Can autism explain objectophila? *Archives of Sexual Behavior, 51*(4), 2117–2133. https://philpapers.org/archive/GATLOC.pdf

Gershoff, E. T. & Font, S. A. (2016). Corporal punishment in U.S. public schools: Prevalence, disparities in use, and status in state and federal policy. *Social Policy Report, 30*(1). https://www.ncbi.nlm.nih.gov/pmc/articles/PMC5766273/.

Ghent, E. (1990). Masochism, submission, surrender: Masochism as a perversion of surrender. *Contemporary Psychoanalysis, 26*(1), 108–136.

Goddard, D. (1972, February 27). The Hell-Fire Club: Visions of debauchery danced in their heads. *The New York Times*. https://www.nytimes.com/1972/02/27/archives/the-hellfire-club-visions-of-debauchery-danced-in-their-heads.html

Goerlich, S. (2020). *The Leather Couch: Clinical Practice with Kinky Clients*. New York, NY: Routledge.

Goerlich, S. (2022). *10,000 Years of Cybersex. Securing Sexuality*. Detroit, MI: The Bound Together Foundation.

Goerlich, S. (2023). *Kink-Affirming Practice: Culturally Competent Therapy from the Leather Chair*. New York, NY: Routledge.

Goerlich, S. (2024). A roomful of leopards: Differentiating intimate partner violence from consensual kink. *Journal of Couple and Family Psychoanalysis*, under review.

GQ India Staff. (2017, August 7). The bizarre reason why genitals are pixelated in Japanese porn. *GQ India*. https://www.gqindia.com/content/japanese-porn-pixelated-genitals-nipples-breasts

Graham, B. C., Butler, S. E., McGraw, R., Cannes, S. M., & Smith, J. (2015). Member perspectives on the role of BDSM communities, *The Journal of Sex Research, 53*(8), 1–15. doi: 10.1080/00224499.2015.1067758

Graham, N. (2014). Polyamory: A call for increased mental health professional awareness. *Archives of Sexual Behavior, 43*(6), 1031–1034. https://doi.org/10.1007/s10508-014-0321-3.

Greitemeyer, T. (2022). Dark personalities and general masochistic tendencies: Their relationships to giving and receiving sexualized pain. *Acta Psychologica, 230* https://doi.org/10.1016/j.actpsy.2022.103715.

Grubbs, J. B. (2020, February 6). Religious, Moral Beliefs May Exacerbate Concerns About Porn Addiction. American Psychological Association. https://www.apa.org/news/press/releases/2020/02/religious-moral-porn-addiction

Habash, G. (2011, February 23). When kindness attacks: A Q&A with Barabara Oakley. *Publishers Weekly*. https://web.p.ebscohost.com/ehost/detail/detail?vid=10&sid=4a8723e7-af98-4a92-885c-ec00221ab1da%40redis&bdata=JnNpdGU9ZWhvc3QtbGl2ZSZzY29wZT1zaXRl#AN=124710784&db=a9h

Hammers, C. (2014). Corporeality: Sadosmasochism and sexual trauma. *Body & Society, 20*(2), 69–90.

Hannigan, B. (2023). *"I Wonder . . .?" The Presence and Implications of Curiosity as a Foundational Ingredient Across Couple and Family Therapy Models*. AURA: Antioch University Repository and Archive. https://aura.antioch.edu/cgi/viewcontent.cgi?article=1963&context=etds

Harris, S. (2023, May 30). An introduction to the fascinating world of predicament bondage. *Kinkly.com*. https://www.kinkly.com/an-introduction-to-the-fascinating-world-of-predicament-bondage/2/17695

Hart, G. & Wellings, K. (2002). Sexual behaviour and its medicalisation: In sickness and in health. *British Medical Journal, 324*(7342), 896–900. https://doi.org/10.1136/bmj.324.7342.896

Hawkinson, K. & Zamboni, B. D. (2014). Adult baby/diaper lovers: An exploratory study of an online community sample. *Archive of Sexual Behavior, 43*(5), 863–77. doi: 10.1007/s10508-013-0241-7. Epub 2014 Jan 29. PMID: 24473941.

Hébert, A. & Weaver, A. (2014). An examination of personality characteristics associated with BDSM orientations. *The Canadian Journal of Human Sexuality, 23*(2), 106–115.

Helfer, E. (2022). *A Kink in the System: Assessing the Impact of Master's Level Human Sexuality Education on Mental Health Practitioners' Attitudes and Perceived Competency Working with Kink-Involved Clients*. [Unpublished doctoral dissertation]. Modern Sex Therapy Institute.

Herbenick, D., Fu, T.C., Wasata, R., & Coleman, E. (2023). Masturbation prevalence, frequency, reasons, and associations with partnered sex in the midst of the COVID-19 pandemic: Findings from a U.S. nationally representative survey. *Archive of Sexual Behavior, 52*(3), 1317–1331. doi: 10.1007/s10508-022-02505-2. Epub 2022 Dec 27. PMID: 36575264; PMCID: PMC9794105.

Hillier, K. M. (2018). Counselling diverse groups: Addressing counsellor bias toward the BDSM and D/S Subculture. *Canadian Journal of Counselling and Psychotherapy, 52*(1), 65–77. Retrieved from https://cjc-rcc.ucalgary.ca/article/view/61095

Holvoet, L., Huys, W., Coppens, V., Seeuws, J., Goethals, K., & Morrens, M. (2017). Fifty shades of Belgian gray: The prevalence of BDSM-related fantasies and activities in the general population. *The Journal of Sexual Medicine, 14*(9), 1152–1159.

Hsu, K. J. & Bailey, J. M. (2019). The "furry" phenomenon: Characterizing sexual orientation, sexual motivation, and erotic target identity inversions in male furries. *Archives of Sexual Behavior, 48*(5), 1349–1369. https://doi.org/10.1007/s10508-018-1303-7

Huang, S., Nyman, T. J., Jern, P., & Santtila, P. (2023). Actual and desired masturbation frequency, sexual distress, and their correlates. *Archives of Sexual Behavior, 52*(7), 3155–3170. doi: 10.1007/s10508-023-02641-3. Epub 2023 Jun 26. PMID: 37365448.

Hughes, S. D. & Hammack, P. L. (2020). Narratives of the origins of kinky sexual desire held by users of a kink-oriented social networking website. *The Journal of Sex Research 59*(3), 360–371, https://doi.org/10.1080/00224499.2020.1840 495.

Human Rights Watch. (2023, July 30). #Outlawed: The Love that Dare Not Speak Its Name. https://features.hrw.org/features/features/lgbt_laws/

Jansen, K., Fried, A., & Chamberlain, J. (2021). An examination of empathy and interpersonal dominance in BDSM practitioners. *The Journal of Sexual Medicine, 18*(3), 549–555. https://doi.org/10.1016/j.jsxm.2020.12.012

Jensen, M. P., Ward, L. C., Thorn, B. E., Ehde, D. M., & Day, M. A. (2017). Measuring the cognitions, emotions, and motivation associated with avoidance behaviors in the context of pain. *The Clinical Journal of Pain, 33*(4), 325–334.

Johns Hopkins University. (2017). Paraphilic Disorders. https://www.hopkinsguides.com/hopkins/view/Johns_Hopkins_Psychiatry_Guide/787119/2.1/Paraphilic_Disorders

Johnson, N. E. & Zhang, K. T. (1991 23(4)). Matriarchy, polyandry, and fertility amongst the Mosuos in China. *Journal of Biosocial Science, 23*(4), 499–505.

Joyal, C. C., Cossette, A., & Lapierre, V. (2015). What exactly is an unusual sexual fantasy? *The Journal of Sexual Medicine 12*(2), 328–340. https://doi.org/10.1111/jsm.12734.

Kabiry, D. M. (2020). Objectum sexuality or objectophilia. In C. Delcea (ed.) *Transtheoretical Approaches to Paraphilic Disorders: Collection from the International Journal of Advanced Studies in Sexology, 2019–2020* (pp. 11–15). Bologna, Italy: Filodiritto.

Kaestle, C. E. & Allen, K. R. (2011). The role of masturbation in healthy sexual development: Perceptions of young adults. *Archives of Sexual Behavior, 40*(5), 983–994. doi: 10.1007/s10508-010-9722-0. Epub 2011 Feb 4. PMID: 21293916.

Karpman, B. The Sexual Psychopath, 42 *J. Crim. L. Criminology & Police Sci. 184*(1951–1952)

Kauffman, M., Silverberg, C., & Odette, F. (2007). *The Ultimate Guide to Sex and Disability.* San Francisco, CA: Cleis Press.

Kekatos, M. (2017, February 13). Fifty shades of HEALTH: Four surprising benefits of kinky sex. *DailyMail.com.* dailymail.co.uk/health/article-4220014/50-shades-HEALTH-suprising-benefits-kinky-sex.html

Kelsey, K., Stiles, B. L., Spiller, L. & Diekhoff, G. M. (2012). Assessment of therapists' attitudes towards BDSM. *Psychology & Sexuality, 4*(3), 255–267. doi: 10.1080/19419899.2012.655255

Kirschbaum, A. & Peterson, Z. (2017). Would you say you "had masturbated" if . . .? The influence of situational and individual factors on labeling a behavior as masturbation. *The Journal of Sex Research, 55*(2), 1–10. 10.1080/00224499.2016.1269307.

Kleinplatz, P. (2006). Learning from extraordinary loves: Lessons from the edge. In P. J. Kleinplatz & C. Moser, *Sadomasochism: Powerful Pleasures* (pp. 325–348). Binghamton, NY: Haworth Press.

Klement, K. R., Sagarin, B. J., & Lee, E. M. (2017). Participating in a culture of consent may be associated with lower rape-supportive beliefs. *The Journal of Sex Research, 54*(1), 130–134.

Kolmes, K., Stock, W., & Moser, C. (2006). Investigating bias in psychotherapy with BDSM clients. *Journal of Homosexuality, 50*(2–3), 301–324. https://doi.org/10.1300/j082v50n02_15.

Langdridge, D. (2007). Speaking the unspeakable: S/M and the eroticization of pain. In D. Langdridge & M. Barker (eds.), *Safe, Sane, and Consensual: Contemporary Perspectives on Sadomasochism* (pp. 85–97). Buffalo, NY: Prometheus Books.

Langdridge, D. & Lawson, J. (2019). The psychology of puppy play: A phenomenological investigation. *Archives of Sexual Behavior, 48*(7), 2201–2215.

Laqueur, T. W. (2004). *Solitary Sex: A cultural history of masturbation.* Zone Books.

Learn, J. R. (2022, November 9). The term 'spirit animal' means more than your favorite animal. *Discover Magazine.* https://www.discovermagazine.com/planet-earth/please-stop-using-the-term-spirit-animal

Lefevre, S. (2012, May). *Compassion, Curiosity, Mindfulness and Flow: The Conditions of Psychotherapists' Positive Experiences of the Therapeutic Process.* The Wright Institute ProQuest Dissertations Publishing. https://www.proquest.com/openview/260a7857401663aea534502fb2ebed21/1?pq-origsite=gscholar&cbl=18750

Lehmiller, J. J. (2018). *Tell Me What You Want: The Science of Sexual Desire and How It Can Help You Improve Your Sex Life.* New York, NY: Da Capo Press.

Lester, P. E., Kohen, I., Stefanacci, R. G., & Feuerman, M. (2016). Sex in nursing homes: A survey of nursing home policies governing resident sexual activity. *Journal of the American Medical Directors Association, 17*(1), 71–74. doi: 10.1016/j.jamda.2015.08.013

Levesque, R. J. (2018). Sadistic personality disorder. In R. L. (ed.), *Encyclopedia of Adolescence* (pp. 3229–3230). New York, NY: Springer International Publishing.

Levy, D. (2007). *Love + Sex with Robots.* New York, NY: HarperCollins.

Ley, D. (2016). *Ethical Porn for Dicks: A Man's Guide to Responsible Viewing Pleasure.* Berkeley, CA: Stonebridge Press.

Li, C., Murad, M., Shahzad, F., Khan, M. A., & Ashraf, S. F. (2020). Dark tetrad personality traits and counterproductive work behavior among doctors in Pakistan. *The International Journal of Health Planning and Management, 35*(5), 1173–1192.

Lilienfeld, S. O., Smith, S. F., & Watts, A. L. (2016). Fearless dominance and its implications for psychopathy: Are the right stuff and the wrong stuff flip sides of the same coin? In V. Zeigler-Hill & D. K. Marcus (eds.), *The Dark Side of Personality: Science and Practice in Social, Personality, and Clinical Psychology* (pp. 65–86). Washington, D.C.: American Psychological Association.

Litam, S. & Speciale, M. (2021). Deconstructing sexual shame: Implications for clinical counselors and counselor educators. *Journal of Counseling Sexology & Sexual Wellness: Research, Practice, and Education, 3*(1), 14–24. 10.34296/03011045.

Lobbestael, J., Slaoui, G., & Gollwitzer, M. (2023). Sadism and personality disorders. *Current Psychiatry Reports, 25*(11), 569–576. doi: 10.1007/s11920-023-01466-0.

Longpre, N., Proulx, J., & Brouillette-Alarie, S. (2016). Convergent validity of three measures of sexual sadism: Value of a dimensional measure. *Sexual Abuse: A Journal of Research and Treatment, 30*(2), 1–17.

Lowrey, A. M. (2004, October 28). From Freud to America: A short history of sadomasochism. *The Harvard Crimson.* https://www.thecrimson.com/article/2004/10/28/from-freud-to-america-a-short/

Lyon, S. (2023, February 20). What to know about ADLs and IADLS. *Very Well Health. com.* https://www.verywellhealth.com/what-are-adls-and-iadls-2510011

Maczkowiack, J. & Schweitzer, R. D. (2018). Postcoital dysphoria: Prevalence and correlates among males. *Journal of Sex & Marital Therapy, 45*(2), 128–140. doi: 10.1080/0092623X.2018.1488326

Marie, C. & Jordan, C. P. (2017, December). Decolonizing Fetish. VisualAids.org. https://visualaids.org/gallery/decolonizing-fetish

Martinez, K. (2016). Somebody's fetish: Self-objectification and body satisfaction among consensual sadomasochists. *Journal of Sex Research, 53*(1), 35–44.

Masuda, K., Ishitobi, Y., Tanaka, Y., & Akiyoshi, J. (2014). Underwear fetishism induced by bilaterally decreased cerebral blood flow in the temporo-occipital lobe. *British Medical Journal Case Reports, bcr201406019.* doi: 10.1136/bcr-2014-206019.

McArthur, N. & Twist, M. L. (2017). The rise of digisexuality: Therapeutic challenges and possibilities. *Sexual and Relationship Therapy, 32*(1), 1–11, https://doi.org/10.1080/14681994.2017.1397950.

McClelland, S. (2012). Measuring sexual quality of life: Ten recommendations for health psychologists. In S. McClelland (ed.), *Handbook of Health Psychology* (pp. 245–267). New York, NY: Taylor & Francis.

McClelland, S. (2014). Intimate justice. In T. Teo (ed.), *Encyclopedia of Critical Psychology* (pp. 1010–1013). London, UK: Springer Reference.

McClelland, S. I. (2010). Intimate justice: A critical analysis of sexual satisfaction. *Social and Personality Psychology Compass, 4*(9), 663–680.

McKee, A., Albury, K., Dunne, M., Grieshaber, S., Hartley, J., Lumby, C., & Matthews, B. (2010). Healthy sexual development: A multidisciplinary framework for research. *International Journal of Sexual Health, 22*(1), 14–19.

McKee, A., Litsou, K., Byron, P., & Ingham, R. (2022). *What Do We Know About the Effects of Porngraphy After Fifty Years of Academic Research?* New York, NY: Routledge.

McManus, M. A., Hargreaves, P., Rainbow, L., & Alison, L. J. (2013). Paraphilias Definition, diagnosis and treatment. *F1000Prime Reports, 5,* 36. https://doi.org/10.12703/P5-36

McNair, B. (2012). *Porno? Chic! How Pornography Changed the World and Made it a Better Place.* New York, NY: Routledge, NY.

Mehdizadeh-Zareanari, A., Ghafarinezhad, A., & Soltani, H. (2013). Fetishism due to methamphetamine (glass) abuse. *Addiction & Health, 51*(1–2), 73–76.

Meibom, J. H. (1650s). *A Treatise of the Use of Flogging in Venereal Affairs: Also of the Office of the Loins and Reins: Written to the Famous Christianus Cassius, Bishop of Lubeck, and Privy-Councellor to the Duke of Holstein.* National Library of Medicine. https://collections.nlm.nih.gov/catalog/nlm:nlmuid-2503037R-bk

Merriam-Webster. (2023, October 17). Protocol. https://www.merriam-webster.com/dictionary/protocol

Meyer, I. H. (2003). Prejudice, social stress, and mental health in lesbian, gay, and bisexual populations: Conceptual issues and research evidence. *Psychological Bulletin, 129*(5), 674–697. https://doi.org/10.1037/0033-2909.129.5.674.

Midori. (2001). *The Seductive Art of Japanese Bondage.* Gardena, CA: Greenery Press.

Mokros, A., Schilling, F., Eher, R., & Nitschke, J. (2012). The Severe Sexual Sadism Scale: Cross-validation and scale properties. *Psychological Assessment, 24*(3), 764–769. doi: 10.1037/a0026419.

Moors, A., Schechinger, H., Balzarini, R., & Flicker, S. (2021). Internalized consensual non-monogamy negativity and relationship quality among people engaged in polyamory, swinging, and open relationships. *Archives of Sexual Behavior, 50*, 1389–1400. https://doi.org/10.1007/s10508-020-01885-7

Moran, M. (2013). DSM to distinguish paraphilias from paraphilic disorders. *Psychiatry Online.* https://psychnews.psychiatryonline.org/doi/full/10.1176/appi.pn.2013.5a19,

Moser, C. (2016). DSM-5 and the paraphilic disorders: Conceptual issues. *Archives of Sexual Behavior, 45*, 2181–2186. https://doi.org/10.1007/s10508-016-0861-9

Moskowitz, C. (2010, July 20). Stone Age carving: Ancient dildo? *LiveScience.* https://www.livescience.com/9971-stone-age-carving-ancient-dildo.html

Murphy, C. & Vess, J. (2003). Subtypes of psychopathy: Proposed differences between narcissistic, borderline, sadistic, and antisocial psychopaths. *Psychiatric Quarterly, 74*(1), 11–29.

National Coalition for Sexual Freedom. (2019). Statement on Consent. https://ncsfreedom.org/wp-content/uploads/2019/12/Consent-Counts-Statement.pdf

National Coalition for Sexual Freedom. (2021). The History of the NCSF. https://ncsfreedom.org/who-we-are/the-history-of-the-ncsf/

National Health Service. (2023, August 8). Why People Self-harm. https://www.nhs.uk/mental-health/feelings-symptoms-behaviours/behaviours/self-harm/why-people-self-harm/

Nevard, I. (2019). Counseling and the kink community: A thematic analysis. *British Journal of Guidance & Counselling, 49*(1), 1–12. https://doi.org/10.1080/03069885.2019.1703899.

Newbold, S. (2023, April 8). Beyond stereotypes: Diving into the world of D/s dynamics. *Progressive Therapeutic.* https://www.progressivetherapeutic.com.au/knowledge-sharing/ds-dynamics.

Newmahr, S. (2010). Power struggles: Pain and authenticity in SM play. *Symbolic Interaction, 33*(3), 389–411. 10.1525/si.2010.33.3.389

Nichols, M. (2011). Psychotherapeutic issues with "kinky" clients: Clinical problems, yours and theirs. In P. Kleinplatz & C. Moser (eds.), *Sadomasochism: Powerful Pleasures* (pp. 281–300). New York, NY: Routledge.

Nin, A. (1992). *Incest: From A Journal of Love. The Unexpurgated Diary of Anais Nin 1932–1934.* New York, NY: Harcourt Books.

Nitschke, J., Osterheider, M., & Mokros, A. (2009). A cumulative scale of severe sexual sadism. *Sexual Abuse, 21*(3), 262–278. doi: 10.1177/1079063209342074.

Nolan, B. (2023, July 18). People are turning to AI chatbots for romantic relationships behind their partners' backs—but many don't consider it cheating. *Business Insider.* https://www.businessinsider.com/replika-ai-romance-behind-partners-backs-cheating-2023-7

Oddie, M. (2022). 'Playing' with race: BDSM, race play, and whiteness in kink. *Panic at the Discourse: An Interdisciplinary Journal, 2*(1), 86–95.

Oneill, T. (2019). *Ungovernable: The Victorian Parent's Guide to Raising Flawless Children.* New York, NY: Little, Brown, and Co.

Oosterhuis, H. (2012). Sexual modernity in the works of Richard von Krafft-Ebing and Albert Moll. *Medical History, 56*(2), 133–155 doi: 10.1017/mdh.2011.30.

Oronowicz, W. & Siwak, M. (2016). Paraphilic infantilism. The analysis of selected cases presented in media with reference to the etiological hypotheses. *Przegląd Seksuologiczny, 4*(48), 10–16.

O'Toole, E. (2015, March 31). This murder in Ireland has made me rethink my sexual practices. *The Guardian.* https://www.theguardian.com/commentisfree/2015/mar/31/murder-ireland-rethink-sexual-practices

Oxford Dictionary (n.d). Authority. oed.com. https://www.oed.com/search/dictionary/?scope=Entries&q=authority

Oyler, L. (2015, August 24). The history of toplessness. *Vice.* https://www.vice.com/en/article/43gy7n/the-history-of-toplessness

Paarnio, M., Sandman, N., Källström, M., Johansson, A., & Jern, P. (2023) The prevalence of BDSM in Finland and the association between BDSM interest and personality traits. *The Journal of Sex Research, 60:4,* 443–451. doi: 10.1080/00224499.2021.2015745

Paasonen, S. (2018). Many splendored things: Sexuality, playfulness, and play. *Sexualities, 21*(4), 537–551. https://doi.org/10.1177/1363460717731928

Paulhus, D. L. & Dutton, D. G. (2016). Everyday sadism. In Z. Ziegler-Hill & D. K. Marcus (eds.), *The Dark Side of Personality: Science and Practice in Social Personality, and Clinical Psychology* (pp. 109–120). Washington, D.C.: American Psychological Association.

Peacock, S. & Patel, S. (2008). Cultural influences on pain. *Reviews in Pain, 1*(2), 6–9

Peasant, C. J. (2014, August). Configurations of Sexual Risk: A Person-Centered Approach. University of Memphis Digital Commons. https://digitalcommons.memphis.edu/cgi/viewcontent.cgi?article=2128&context=etd

Pettyjohn, M. E., Tseng, C. F., & Blow, A. J. (2020). Therapeutic utility of discussing therapist/client intersectionality in treatment: When and how? *Family Process, 59*(2), 313–327. https://doi.org/10.1111/famp.12471

Phillips, J. (2005). *How to Read Sade*. New York, NY: W.W. Norton and Co.

Phillips, J., Ainslie, S., Fowler, A., & Westaby, C. (2022, July). Putting Professional Curiosity into Practice. Her Majesty's Inspectorate of Probation. https://shura. shu.ac.uk/30544/1/Phillips-PuttingProfessionalPractice%28VoR%29.pdf

Pittagora, D. (2015, March 19). The intersection of gender roles and BDSM power roles. *Manhattan Alternative.* https://www.manhattanalternative.com/ the-intersection-of-gender-roles-and-bdsm-power-roles

Podolan, M. & Gelo, O. C. (2023). The functions of safety in psychotherapy: An integrative theoretical perspective across therapeutic schools. *Clinical Neuropsychiatry, 20*(3), 193–204.

Price, M. (2023, January 9). Sexual bondage date turned deadly when victim bit man's genitals, Florida cops say. *Miami Herald.* https://www.miamiherald. com/news/state/florida/article270910772.html

Price, T. J. & Gold, M. S. (2018). From mechanism to cure: Renewing the goal to eliminate the disease of pain. *Pain Medicine, 19*(8), 1525–1549.

Prottle, Z. (2023, October 19). 10 Most Common Addictions. Addiction Center. https://www.addictioncenter.com/addiction/10-most-common-addictions/

Regnerus, M., Price, J., & Gordon, D. (2017). Masturbation and partnered sex: Substitutes or complements? *Archives of Sexual Behavior, 46*(7), 2111–2121. doi: 10.1007/s10508-017-0975-8. Epub 2017 Mar 24. PMID: 28341933.

Rehor, J. E. (2015). Sensual, erotic, and sexual behaviors of women from the "kink" community. *Archives of Sexual Behavior, 44*(4), 825–36. doi: 10.1007/s10508-015-0524-2. Epub 2015 Mar 21. PMID: 25795531; PMCID: PMC4379392.

Richardson, K. (2015). The Asymmetrical 'Relationship': Parallels between Prostitution and the Development of Sex Robots. Campaign Against Sex Robots. https://campaignagainstsexrobots.org/papers/

Richters, J., DeVisser, R. O., Rissel, C. E., Grulich, A. E., & Smith, A. M. (2008). Demographic and psychosocial features of participants in bondage and discipline, "sadomasochism" or dominance and submission (BDSM): Data from a national survey. *The Journal of Sexual Medicine, 5*(7), 1660–1668.

Rowland, D. L., Hevesi, K., Conway, G. R., & Kolba, T. N. (2020). Relationship between masturbation and partnered sex in women: Does the former facilitate, inhibit, or not affect the latter? *Journal of Sexual Medicine, 17*(1), 37–47. doi: 10.1016/j.jsxm.2019.10.012. Epub 2019 Nov 21. PMID: 31759932.

Rubin, G. (1992). Thinking sex: Notes for a radical theory of the politics of sexuality. In C. Vance (ed.), *Pleasure and Danger: Exploring Female Sexuality* (pp. 267–319). Pandora/Harper Collins.

Rubin, G. (2012). *Thinking Sex: Notes for a Radical Theory of Politics of Sexuality*. Durham, NC: Duke University Press.

Rubin, L. (2021). Stefani Goerlich on Becoming a Kink-Affirming Therapist. Psychotherapy.net. https://www.psychotherapy.net/interview/stefani-goerlich-becoming-kink-affirming-therapist,

Rulof, P. (2011). *Ageplay: From Diapers to Diplomas.* Las Vegas, NA: The Naxca Plains Corporation.

Sagarin, B. (2013). Lecture on hormones, pain, and altered states: A scientific search for the essence of sadomasochism. *Personal Collection of B. Sagarin,* Northern Illinois University of Dekalb, IL.

Sagarin, B. J., Cutler, B., Cutler, N., Lawler-Sagarin, K. A., & Matuszewich, L. (2009). Hormonal changes and couple bonding in consensual sadomasochistic activity. *Archives of Sexual Behavior 38*(2), 186–200. DOI 10.1007/s10508–008–9374–5.

Sagarin, B. J., Lee, E. M., & Klement, K. R. (2015). Sadomasochism without sex? Exploring the parallels between BDSM and extreme rituals. *Journal of Positive Sexuality, 1,* 50–55. http://journalofpositivesexuality.org/wp-content/uploads/2016/05/Parallels-Between-BDSM-and-Extreme-Ritual-Sagarin-Lee-Klement.pdf.

Saketopoulou, A. (2023). *Sexuality Beyond Consent: Risk, Race, and Traumatophilia.* New York, NY: NYU Press.

Salmon, L. (2017). The four questions: A framework for integrating an understanding of oppression dynamics in clinical work and supervision. In: R. Allan & S. Singh Poulsen (eds.) *Creating Cultural Safety in Couple and Family Therapy.* AFTA Springer Briefs in Family Therapy. Cham: Springer. https://doi.org/10.1007/978-3-319-64617-6_2

Sand, L. (2019). Removing judgement: Discussing BDSM in adult sexuality education. *American Journal of Sexuality Education, 14*(2), 258–267.

Sandnabba, N. K., Santtila, P., Alison, L., & Nordling, N. (2002). Demographics, sexual behaviour, family background and abuse experiences of practitioners of sadomasochistic sex: A review of recent research. *Sexual and Relationship Therapy, 17*(1), 39–55.

Schnider, A. (2012). Confabulation and reality filtering. In V. Ramachandran (ed.), *Encyclopedia of Human Behavior,* 2nd Edition (pp. 563–571). Amsterdam, Netherlands: Elsevier Inc. https://www.sciencedirect.com/topics/nursing-and-health-professions/disorientation

Schori, A., Jackowski, C., & Schön, C. (2022). How safe is BDSM? A literature review on fatal outcome in BDSM play. *International Journal of Legal Medicine, 136*(1), 287–295. 10.1007/s00414–021–02674–0.

Science of BDSM. (2024). About the Team. https://scienceofbdsm.com/about-the-team

Scorolli, C., Ghirlanda, S., Enquist, M., Zattoni, S., & Jannini, E. (2007). Relative prevalence of different fetishes. *International Journal of Impotence Research, 19*(4) 432–437. DOI: 10.1038/sj.ijir.3901547.

Scott, C. (2015). *Thinking Kink: The Collision of BDSM, Feminism, and Popular Culture.* Jefferson, NC: McFarland & Company, Inc.

Seham, A. (2001). *Whose Improv Is It Anyway?* Jackson, MS: University Press of Mississippi.

Sheff, E. (2014). The 7 different kinds of non-monogamy. *Psychology Today.* https://www.psychologytoday.com/us/blog/the-polyamorists-next-door/201407/7-different-kinds-non-monogamy.

Sheppard, E. (2020). Chronic pain as emotion. *Journal of Literary & Cultural Disability Studies, 14*(1), 5–20. https://doi.org/10.3828/jlcds.2019.17.

Shields, L. B. & Hunsaker III, J. (2020). Autoerotic asphyxiation. In B. Madea (ed.), *Asphyxiation, Suffocation, and Neck Pressure Deaths* (pp. 285–292). New York, NY: Routledge. DOI: 10.1201/9780429188947-28.

Shorter, E. (2014). Sexual Sunday school: The DSM and the gatekeeping of morality. *Virtual Mentor, 16*(11), 932–937. doi: 10.1001/virtualmentor.2014.16.11. mhst1-1411. PMID: 25397655.

Shulman, J.L. & Horne, S.G. (2003). The use of self-pleasure: Masturbation and body image among African-American and European-American women. *Psychology of Women Quarterly, 27*(3), 262–269. https://doi.org/10.1111/1471-6402.00106

Sicart, Miquel. (2014). *Play Matters.* Cambridge, MA: MIT Press.

Silva, A. & Mercury, K. (2015). *Through Pain, More Gain? A Survey into the Psychosocial Benefits of Sadomasochism* [Thesis]. *Figshare.* https://doi.org/10.6084/m9.figshare.12283853.v1

Simone, M (2022, August 8). What is age regression and how can you overcome it? *PsychCentral.* From https://psychcentral.com/pro/are-you-emotionally-regressing

Simula, B. L. (2019). Pleasure, power, and pain: A review of the literature on the experiences of BDSM participants. *Sociology Compass, 13,* e12668. https://doi.org/10.1111/soc4.12668

Slagstad, K. (2023). Visualizing BDSM and AIDS activism: Archiving pleasures, sanitizing history. *Journal of the History of Medicine and Allied Sciences, 78*(3), 270–303. https://doi.org/10.1093/jhmas/jrad012.

Sloan, K. (2019). BDSM is the new rape myth. *Herizons, 40.*

Song, X., Xu, B., & Zhao, Z. (2022). Can people experience romantic love for artificial intelligence? An empirical study of intelligent assistants. *Information & Management, 59*(2), https://doi.org/10.1016/j.im.2022.103595.

Sprott, R.A., Herbitter, C., Grant, P., Moser, C., & Kleinplatz, P.J. (2023) Clinical guidelines for working with clients involved in kink. *Journal of Sex & Marital Therapy, 49*(8), 978–995. DOI: 10.1080/0092623X.2023.2232801

Sprott, R. A. & Randall, A. (2016). Black and blues: Sub drop, top drop, event drop, and scene drop. *Journal of Positive Sexuality, 2*(3), 53–61.

Sprott, R. A. & Williams, D. J. (2019). Is BDSM a sexual orientation or serious leisure? *Current Sexual Health Reports, 11*(2), 75–79.

Stein, S. D. (2000). Safe Sane Consensual. LeatherLeadership.org. https://www.leatherleadership.org/library/safesanestein.htm

Steinmetz, C. & Maginn, P. (2014). The landscape of BDSM venues. In: C. Steinmetz & P. Maginn (eds.) *(Sub-)urban Sexscapes: Geographies and Regulation of the Sex Industry* (pp. 117–138). London: Routledge.

Stevenson, D. (2001). *The Beggar's Benison: Sex Clubs of Enlightenment Scotland and Their Rituals*. East Lothian, Scotland: Tuckwell Press.

Stromberg, J. (2013, November 22). The neuroscientist who discovered he was a psychopath. *Smithsonian Magazine*. https://www.smithsonianmag.com/science-nature/the-neuroscientist-who-discovered-he-was-a-psycho-path-180947814/

Swartzendruber, A. & Zenilman, J. M. (2010). A national strategy to improve sexual health. *Journal of the American Medical Association, 304*(9), 1005–1006. http://dx.doi.org/10.1001/jama.2010.1252

Switch, G. (2018, February 8). *RACK: Risk Aware Consensual Kink Challenging Absolutism; A Framework of Risk Acknowledgement*. (A. O. Nomis, Interviewer).

TASHRA. (2023). *Playing with Dark Emotions: Playing with Fear and Shame in Scenes of Humiliation, Objectification, and Dehumanization*. San Francisco, CA: TASHRA.

TASHRA. (2024). Our Story. https://tashra.org/our-story/

Tatum, A. K. & Niedermeyer, T. (2021). Shining a light in the dungeon: A content analysis of sexual and gender minority representation in the kink literature. *Psychology of Sexual Orientation and Gender Diversity, 8*(3), 328–343.

Tiidenberg, K. & Paasonen, S. (2019). Littles: Affects and aesthetics in sexual age-play. *Sexuality & Culture, 23*(2), 375–393. https://doi.org/10.1007/s12119-018-09580-5

Toth, J. (2015). *Perverse Psychology: The Pathologization of Sexual Violence and Transgenderism*. London, UK: Routledge.

Townsend, E., Ness, J., Waters, K., Kapur, N., Turnbull, P., Cooper, J., & Hawton, K. (2015). Self-harm and life problems: Findings from the multicentre study of self-harm in England. *Social Psychiatry and Psychiatric Epidemiology, 51*(2), 183–192.

Trammell, A. (2020). Torture, play, and the Black experience. *Game: The Italian Journal of Game Studies, 8*(9), 33–49. https://www.gamejournal.it/torture-play/.

Tupper, P. (2016). *Our Lives, Our History: Consensual Master/Slave Relationships from Ancient Times to the 21st Century*. Brooklyn, NY: Perfectbound Press.

Turley, E. (2016). Like nothing I've ever felt before: Understanding consensual BDSM as embodied experience. *Psychology & Sexuality, 7*(2), 149–162.

Turley, E. (2018). Leading and following? Understanding the power dynamics in consensual BDSM. In J. K. Beggan & S. T. Allison (eds.) *Leadership and Sexuality*. Cheltenham: Elgar Online.

Turvey, B. E. (2012). Pathological altruism: Victims and motivational types. In B. Oakley, A. Knafo, G. Madhavan, & D. S. Wilson (eds.), *Pathological Altruism* (pp. 177–192). Oxford, UK/New York, NY: Oxford University Press.

Udodiong, I. (2019, October 21). Meet the naked tribes of Nigeria—where people wear leaves and little to nothing. *Pulse*. https://www.pulse.ng/bi/lifestyle/meet-the-naked-tribes-of-nigeria-where-people-wear-leaves-and-little-to-nothing/w3ttqxv van der Beek, S. & Thomas, L. (2023). "I wish people knew that there are other flavors": Reflections on the representation of poly-kink in mainstream media by polyamorous kinksters in the Netherlands. *Sexualities, 0*(0), 1–20. https://doi.org/10.1177/13634607231152601

Vandiver, D. & Braithwaite, J. (2022). *Sex Crimes: Research and Realities.* New York, NY: Routledge.

Victoria Department of Health. (2023, February 17). Dissociation and Dissociative Disorders. BetterHealth. https://www.betterhealth.vic.gov.au/health/conditionsandtreatments/dissociation-and-dissociative-disorders

Vilkin, E. & Sprott, R. (2021). Consensual non-monogamy among kink-identified adults: Characteristics, relationship experiences, and unique motivations for polyamory and open relationships. *Archives of Sexual Behavior, 50*(4), 1521–1536. doi: 10.1007/s10508-021-02004-w. Epub 2021 Jun 14. PMID: 34128141.

Waldura, J. F., Arora, I., Randall, A. M., Farala, J. P., & Sprott, R. A. (2016). Fifty shades of stigma: Exploring the health care experiences of kink-oriented patients. *Journal of Sexual Medicine, 13*(12), 1918–1929. https://doi.org/10.1016/j.jsxm.2016.09.019

Walsh, A. (2000). Improve and care: Responding to inappropriate masturbation in people with severe intellectual disabilities. *Sexuality and Disability, 18*(1), 27–39. doi: 10.1023/A:1005473611224.

Watts-Jones, D. (2010). Location of self: Opening the door to dialogue on intersectionality in the therapy process. *Family Process, 49*(3), 405–420. https://doi.org/10.1111/j.1545-5300.2010.01330.x

Webster, C. & Klaserner, M. (2019). Fifty shades of socializing: Slosh and munch events in the BDSM community. *Event Management, 23*(1), 135–147. https://doi.org/10.3727/152599518X15378845225401

Weisel-Barth, J. (2013). The fetish in Nicole Krauss' Great House and in clinical practice. *Psychoanalytic Dialogues, 23*(2), 180–186.

Weisman, C. (2023, May 4). How common is BDSM sex? Very. In fact, you've probably done it. *Fatherly.* https://www.fatherly.com/life/bdsm-kinky-sex-not-uncommon

Weiss, M. D. (2006). Working at play: BDSM sexuality in the San Francisco Bay area. *Anthropologica, 48*(2), 229–245.

Westen, D., Blagov, P. S., Harenski, K., Kilts, C., & Hamann, S. (2006). The neural basis of motivated reasoning: An fMRI study of emotional constraints on political judgement. *Journal of Cognitive Neuroscience, 18*(11), 1947–1958.

Wertheimer, A. (2003). *Consent to Sexual Relations.* Cambridge: Cambridge University Press.

Wiech, K. & Tracey, I. (2013). Pain, decisions, and actions: A motivational perspective. *Frontiers in Neuroscience, 7*(46), https://doi.org/10.3389/fnins.2013.00046.

Wignall, L. (2023). The role of the Internet in research on BDSM. In B. Simula, R. Bauer, & L. Wignall (eds.) *The Power of BDSM: Play, Communities, and Consent in the 21st Century.* New York, NY: Oxford Academic.

Wignall, L., McCormack, M., Cook, T., & Jaspal, R. (2022). Findings from a community survey of individuals who engage in pup play. *Archives of Sexual Behavior, 51*(1), 1–10. 10.1007/s10508–021–02225-z.

Williams, D., Thomas, J. N., Prior, E. A., & Christensen, M. C. (2014). From "SSC" and "RACK" to the "4cs": Introducing a new framework for negotiating BDSM participation. *Electronic Journal of Human Sexuality, 17*.

Wiseman, J. (2000). *Jay Wiseman's Erotic Bondage Handbook*. Gardena, CA: Greenery Press.

Wismeijer, A. A. & van Assen, M. A. (2013). Psychological characteristics of BDSM practitioners. *The Journal of Sexual Medicine, 10*(8), 1943–1952.

World Health Organization. (2011). Sexual and Reproductive Health: Core Competencies in Primary Care. https://www.who.int/reproductivehealth/publications/health_systems/9789241501002/en/

Worthen, M. G. (2022). *Sexual Deviance and Society: A Sociological Examination*. New York, NY: Routledge.

Wright, S. (2010). Depathologizing consensual sexual sadism, sexual masochism, transvestic fetishism, and fetishism. *Archives of Sexual Behavior, 39*(6), 1229–1230. DOI: 10.1007/s10508-010-9651-y.

Wright, S., Bowling, J., McCabe, S., Benson, J. K., Stambaugh, R., & Cramer, R. J. (2022). Sexual violence and nonconsensual experiences among alt-sex communities' members. *Journal of Interpersonal Violence, 37*(23–24). https://doi.org/10.1177/08862605211062999

Xygalatas, D., Mitkidis, P., Fischer, R., Reddish, P., Skewes, J., Geertz, A. W., Roepstorff, A., & Bulbulia, J. (2013). Extreme rituals promote prosociality. *Psychological Science, 24*(8), 1602–1605. https://doi.org/10.1177/0956797612472910

Yager, J., Kay, J., & Kelsay, K. (2021). Clinicians' cognitive and affective biases and the practice of psychotherapy. *American Journal of Psychotherapy, 74*(3), 119–126.

Yakeley, J. & Wood, H. (2014). Paraphilias and paraphilic disorders: Diagnosis, assessment, and management. *Advances in Psychiatric Treatment, 20*(3), 202–213. doi:10.1192/apt.bp.113.011197.

Yost, M. R. & Hunter, L. E. (2012). BDSM practitioners' understandings of their initial attraction to BDSM sexuality: Essentialist and constructivist narratives. *Psychology & Sexuality, 3*(3), 244–259.

Zambelli, L. (2017). Subcultures, narratives, and identification: An empirical study of BDSM (bondage and discipline, domination and submission, sadism and masochism) practices in Italy. *Sexuality and Culture, 21*(2), 471–492. doi: 10.1007/s12119-016-9400-z.

Zamboni, B. (2017). Characteristics of subgroups in the adult baby/diaper lover community. *Journal of Sexual Medicine, 14*(11), 1421–1429.

INDEX

Abel, G. G. 92, 96
activities for daily living (ADLs) 171
addiction 138, 155; *see also*
    problematic sexual behavior
adult babies/diaper lovers (ABDLs)
    82–4, 92; *see also* caregiver kinks
Afana, E. D. 71
aftercare 120–3, 170
age play 78–84
Age Play (Rulof) 78
agency: authority exchange and 38;
    history of kink culture and 12;
    kink-affirming risk assessment and
    158–9, 160; punishments and 32;
    safety and risks and 155
aggressive play 153
AIDS crisis 11, 163–4
alcohol intoxication 34, 49, 173;
    see also substance use
Alegre, S. M. 101
algolagnic disorders 145
Allen, K. R. 131
Allendar, D. B. 184
Alternative Sexualities Health
    Research Alliance (TASHRA)
    106, *107*
Ambler, J. K. 70

American Law Institute 186–7
American Sexual Revolution in the
    1960s 127
anomalous sexual preferences 146
anomalous target preferences 145–6
anonymous sexual preferences 145
Ansara, Y. G. 120
antisocial personality disorder 65–6,
    72–4
anxiety 50, 137
APA Dictionary 85
appearance, control over 40–1
Arnaud, S. 97
artificial intelligence (AI) 98,
    99–100, 101–2
Artsy Editorial 3
asphyxia 33–4, 49
assessment: antisocial personalities
    and 73; empathetic sadism and
    61; fetishes and fetishistic desire
    and 100; kink-affirming risk
    assessment 158–63; masochistic
    altruism and 69–70; risk
    assessment 100, 158–63, 169–73;
    risk assessment checklist 169–73;
    sadomasochism and 59–60, 61,
    63–5, 69–70, 73, 76

attachment: dominance and submission and 43; fetishes and fetishistic desire and 95, 96; risk assessment checklist 171; sadism spectrum and 66

attachment disorders 97

authenticity 38, 50

authority exchange 5, 23–4, 36–8, 49–51; *see also* discipline; dominance; submission

authority reinforcement 31–2

authority transfer 36–7

autoerotic asphyxiation 33–4, 49

auto-erotic bondage 33–4; *see also* bondage

autonomy 12, 158–9, 160

aversion 53–4

avoidance 53–4

babies, adult *see* adult babies/diaper lovers (ABDLs)

Baggett, R. L. 184

Barber, T. 97–8

Barker, E. D. 51

Bastian, B. 56, 74

bathroom/toilet control 40

Bauer, R. 48, 78, 80

Baumeister, R. F. 6, 68–9, 74

BDSM in general 4–5, 9–11, 157

Bedbible Research Center 92

bedroom bondage 17–8; *see also* bondage

Beech, A. R. 141, 143, 145, 146

Beggar's Bennison 10

behavior, control of 15; *see also* control

behavior modification 31

behavioral fetishes 91; *see also* fetishes and fetishistic desire

Behind the Green Door 11

benefits: authority exchange and 49–51; BDSM play and 69; fetishes and 90, 100–2; masturbation and 132–3; pain and

54–5, 68, 74–6; risk assessment and 153, 158; roleplay and 87–8; rules and 24

Bentham, J. 52, 53

Berger, P. 73

Berry, M. D. 183, 184

bestiality, compared to pet play 84–5

Bhadelia, A. 53

bias: history of clinical biases 124–7; kink-affirming treatment and 160–2, 181, 188–9; overview 12; pain versus sensation and 67–8

Big Five personality traits 6–7, 43–4

BIPOC community 6, 12–3, 179–80

Black, L. L. 176, 177

bodily autonomy 12; *see also* autonomy

body awareness 74

body confidence 74

body fetishes 91; *see also* fetishes and fetishistic desire

bondage: mechanical bondage 19–21; overview 4–5, 15, 16–22; predicament play 22; ropes and restraints 17–9; safety and risks and 33–5

Borzarth, J. D. 160

The Bottoming Book (Hardy & Easton) 9

bottoms 22, 45–9, 153

boundaries: 4Ps model and 169; masturbation and 133–4; punishments and 30–1; risk assessment and 158, 172; rules and 24; sadomasochism and 70; safety and risks and 153–4; variations on D/s dynamics and 46

Bowman, C. P. 132

Braithwaite, J. 66, 73

bratting 32

Braun-Harvey, D. 147, 148–49, 151

Breithaupt, F. 60–2

Brennan, F. 67

Brown, A. 128, 140

Brown, B. 75
Brown, J. 178
Buaban, J. 132
Buckels, E. E. 62
Bullough, V. 132
Byron, P. 135, 136

Camacho, N. A. 2
caregiver kinks 78–84
caregiver role 80–1; *see also* age play; caregiver kinks
Carlström, C. 50, 104, 105
Carvalheira, A. 131
cathartic relief 74
caution 167–8
Center for Positive Sexuality 167–8
chains 16, 17–8; *see also* bondage
Charleston, L. 2
cheating 138
choice 22, 32, 160
chronic pain 56; *see also* pain
Cito, G. 131
Clark-Flory, T. 72
Cleveland Clinic 132
client-centered therapy 159–60
clinicians 178–82; *see also* kink-affirming treatment
clothing control 41
coercive paraphilic disorder 72
coercive play 153
cognitive schemes 66
cognitive-affective control 55
Coleman, E. 131
collaring/consideration ceremonies 26; *see also* rituals
communication: debriefing and 122–3; importance of 39; non-monogamy and 140; relationship skills and 155–6; sadomasochism and 74; safety and risks and 156; total power exchange (TPE) and 42; *see also* negotiation
community 86, 163–9; *see also* kink community

Community-Academic Consortium for Research on Alternative Sexualities (CARAS) 108, *109*
compassion 162–3
compulsive behaviors 149–51, 172; *see also* problematic sexual behavior
confidentiality 158
conflict resolution 32, 155–6; *see also* communication
connection: aftercare and 120–3; authority exchange and 50; fetishes and fetishistic desire and 93; pet play and 86; purposeful pain and 55, 57; risk assessment checklist 172
Connolly, P. 6
consensual non-consent 76; *see also* consent
consensual non-monogamy *see* consent; ethical non-monogamy
consent: aftercare and 120; criminal behaviors and 147; exhibitionistic disorder and 146; explicit prior permission 148, 186–7; 4Cs model and 167–8; FRIES ("Freely given," "Reversible," "Informed," "Enthusiastic," "Specific") and 166–7; Kink Clinical Guidelines and 181; kink demographics and 9; legal issues and 184–8; overview 4; paraphilias and 143–4; pornography and 135–6; principles of responsible sexual behavior and 149; punishments and 32; RACK (Risk-Aware, Consensual Kink) and 164–6; risk assessment checklist 170, 173; sadomasochism and 70; safety and risks and 152, 154, 155; SSC (safe, sane, and consensual) and 164; total power exchange (TPE) and 39–43; variations on D/s dynamics and 46; voyeuristic

disorder and 146; when sexual behaviors are a problem 147–8; *see also* negotiation
consistency 32
Constantinides, D. 184
continuing education 101
control: authority exchange and 37–8; cultural factors and 13–4; discipline and 23; exchange of 5, 15, 39–42; 4Ps model and 168–9; kink-affirming risk assessment and 159; in the treatment room 175–8; variations on D/s dynamics and 46; *see also* bondage; discipline
Coppens, V. 6
coprophilia (feces fetish) 83, 146
corporal punishment 4, 15, 23; *see also* discipline; punishments
courtship disorders 146
Cowart, L. 54
Cox, D. 128
criminal behaviors: antisocial personalities and 72–3; legal issues and 185–8; paraphilias and 142–4, 147; pedophilic disorder and 145; risk assessment checklist 173; *see also* legal factors
Crimmins, J. E. 53
cross-dressing 145
Cruz, A. 12
Csillag, V. 61
cuckolding 89–90; *see also* fetishes and fetishistic desire
cultural factors: everyday sadism and 63; fetishes and fetishistic desire and 89, 93–4, 96; idea of pain and 53–4; masturbation and 131, 131–2; overview 12–4; pain and 66–67; purposeful pain and 57; rituals and 24–5; therapeutic context and 176–7; what counts as normal 128; *see also* Time+Place idea
Cumberpatch, C. 94
curiosity 162–3

daily functioning 135, 171–2
Damm, C. 74
Dancer 39
Dashwood, F. 10
Davis-Stober, C. P. 34
de Brosses, C. 93–4
De Neef, N. 6
de Sade, M. 52, 59, 62–3, 66, 126
death 49
debriefing 122–3; *see also* aftercare
decision control 40
decorative bondage 16
deep consent 168; *see also* consent
Deep Throat 11
degradation play 153
Delcea, C. 100
demographics, kink 5–9, **7–8**, 92
depression 50, 137
Deri, J. 48
desire 129–30
diagnosis: antisocial personalities 72–4; differential diagnostics 68–74; Kink Clinical Guidelines and 183–4; kink-affirming treatment and 192; paraphilias and the DSM and 140–7; pathological altruism 67–70; sadism spectrum and 57–9, 60, 63–4; sadistic personality disorder (SPD) and 65–6; self-harm 70–2; *see also* kink-affirming treatment; mental illness
Diagnostic and Statistical Manual of Mental Disorders (DSM): antisocial personalities and 72, 73, 74; distress and 148; history of clinical biases and 127; paraphilias and 140–7, *143*; sadism spectrum and 57–9; sadistic personality disorder (SPD) and 65–6, 72, 73; sexual sadism disorder and 63–4
diaper lovers 82–4, 92; *see also* caregiver kinks
differential diagnostics 68–74, 192; *see also* diagnosis

digisexuality 97–99, 101–2; *see also* fetishes and fetishistic desire

disabilities, people with 56, 179–80

disapproval 53–4

discipline: overview 4–5, 15, 23–32; predicament play and 22; protocols 27–9; punishments 29–32; rituals 24–7; rules 23–4; safety and risks and 33–5

disconnection 50; *see also* connection

discrimination: history of clinical biases 124–7; Kink Clinical Guidelines and 181; overview 72; roleplay and 88

disease 118–9, 150

disease model 149

dissociation/disorientation 171–2

distress 147–8, 151, 173; *see also* guilt; shame

domestic violence *see* intimate partner violence

dominance: adult babies/diaper lovers and 84; authority exchange 36–8; overview 4–5; personality traits and 43–5; power exchange and 38–43; risks and benefits of authority exchange and 49–51; variations on D/s dynamics 45–9

Dominants: authority exchange and 37–8; kink demographics and 6; rituals and 25–6; self-bondage and 19; total power exchange (TPE) and 38–43; variations on D/s dynamics 45–9

Doniger 125

Drouin, M. 49

drug intoxication 49, 173; *see also* substance use

D/s dynamics 45–9; *see also* dominance; Dominants; submission; submissives

Dunn, B. 72

Dutton, D. G. 58

dysregulated sexual behavior 149–51; *see also* problematic sexual behavior

Earl, J. E. 90

Easton, D. 9, 51, 152

educational opportunities: overview 104–9; research/educational organizations 106–9; risk assessment checklist 172; safety and risks and 153, 156; skill-building education 35, 105; virtual opportunities 109–10; *see also* kink community

Elders, J. 2

emotional risks 117–8; *see also* risks

empathetic sadism 60–2; *see also* sadism

empathy 55, 162–3

empowerment 160

environmental factors 66

equality 9–10, 12

Erickson, J. M. 62

erotic asphyxiation 33–4, 49

erotica 3–4, 9

ethical hedonism 53

ethical non-monogamy 6, 138–40

Eusei, D. 100

evening rituals 25; *see also* rituals

events *see* kink community

everyday sadism *see* sadism

exercise control 41

exhibitionism 146, 173

Exit to Eden (Roquelaure) 11

expectations 24, 27–8

explicit prior permission 148, 187; *see also* consent; negotiation

Fahs, B. 132

family: Kink Clinical Guidelines and 181; risk assessment checklist 171, 172; rituals and 24

farm animals, pet play and 87

fatal outcomes 49

fearless dominance 73–4
Felluga, D. F. 94
feminist perspective 56
fetishes and fetishistic desire: common fetishes 92–3; digisexuality 97–100; history of kink culture and 9–12, 93–5; mental illness and 95–6; objectophilia 96–7; overview 89–92; risks and benefits 100–2; Time+Place idea and 3
fetishistic disorder 145
Fifty Shades of Grey books 11, 59
financial control 40
Font, S. A. 4
food control 41
Fors, M. 175–6
4Cs model 167–8
4Ps model 168–9
Frank, E. 132
Frankfurther, D. 93
Franklin, B. 10
Frayn, D. 161
Freud, S. 94–5, 126–7
FRIES ("Freely given," "Reversible," "Informed," "Enthusiastic," "Specific") 166–7, 168
frotteuristic disorder 146
frustration tolerance 155–6
functional impairment 146–7, 148, 151, 171–2
furry community 85

gags 15; *see also* bondage
Gatzia, D. E. 97
Gay Male S/M Activists (GMSMA) 164
gay military veterans 10–1; *see also* LGBTQIA+ community
Gelo, O. C. 158, 159
gender 177, 181, 183
general time control 42
Gershoff, E. T. 4
Ghent, E. 68
goals/intentions 113–4

Goddard, D. 10
Goerlich, S. 6, 13, 60, 69, 83, 99, 161, 162, 168–9, 178, 179, 183–4
Gold, M. S. 67
Golden Age of Porn 11
GQ India Staff 3
Graham, B. C. 110
Graham, N. 188
greetings and farewell protocols 27
Greitemeyer, T. 58
Grubbs, J. B. 138
guilt: masturbation and 132, 135, 136; paraphilic disorders and 145; pornography and 136; sadomasochism and 69; safety and risks 154–5

Habash, G. 69
Hammack, P. L. 6
Hammers, C. 74
Hannigan, B. 162
hard bondage 17–8; *see also* bondage
Hardy, J. 9, 51, 152
Hare Psychopathy checklist tool 73–4
Harkins 145
harm reduction strategies 11, **163**–4
harm to others 147–8; *see also* problematic sexual behavior
Harris, S. 22
Hart, G. 125
Hawkinson, K. 83, 84
health risks: masturbation and 131; negotiation and 117–8; principles of responsible sexual behavior and 150; STI, disease, and pregnancy protection and 118–9; *see also* risks
Healthy Sexual Development (McKee) 152
hedonism 53
Helfer, E. 178
Hellfire Club 10, 11
Herbenick, D. 132
heroism 73

hierarchical connections: authority exchange and 36; punishments and 31–2; total power exchange (TPE) and 39; variations on D/s dynamics and 47

Hillier, K. M. 140

Hirschfeld 95

His Porn, Her Pain (Klein) 136–7

The History and Arts of the Dominatrix (Nomis) 124

history of kink culture: bondage and 17; fetishes and fetishistic desire 93–5; history of clinical biases 124–7; kink culture 9–12; kink-affirming treatment and 192; masturbation 131–2; overview 2–3; paraphilias and the DSM and 141–2; sadomasochism 52; Time+Place idea and 2–4

Holvoet, L. 6

homosexuality 3; *see also* LGBTQIA+ community

honesty 150

honorifics use protocols 28

Horne, S. G. 131

How to Build a Sex Room show 11–2

Huang, S. 132, 134

Hughes, S. D. 6

Human Rights Watch 3

humiliation play 153

Hunter, L. E. 6

Hurts So Good (Cowart) 54

Huys, W. 6

hypersexuality 149–51; *see also* problematic sexual behavior

idea fetishes 89–90, 91–2; *see also* fetishes and fetishistic desire

identity: digisexuality and 98; Kink Clinical Guidelines and 180; kink-affirming treatment and 188–9; pet play and 86; purposeful pain and 55; risk assessment checklist

172; rituals and 25; variations on D/s dynamics and 45–9

illegal activities: legal issues and 184–8; paraphilias and 142–4, 147; pedophilic disorder and 145; risk assessment checklist 173

imaginative power exchange: caregiver kinks 78–84; overview 77; pet play 84–7; risks and benefits 87–8; *see also* power and power exchange; roleplay

impairment 146–7, 148, 151

inanimate objects *see* object fetishes

infants, adult 82–4, 92; *see also* caregiver kinks

informed consent 159

Ingham, R. 135, 136

injury: aftercare and 122; authority exchange and 49; masturbation and 133; risk assessment checklist 170; *see also* risks; safety

instrumental activities of daily living (IADLs) 171

instruments 116–7

intent 113–4

International Classification of Diseases, Tenth Edition (ICD-10) 58, 73

interpersonal bonding 55, 57

interracial relationships 10

intersectionality: Kink Clinical Guidelines and 180; purposeful pain and 56; therapeutic context and 176–7

interventions 182–4

intimate justice 2, 155

intimate partner violence 72, 168–9, 181

intoxication 34, 49, 50; *see also* substance use

Jansen, K. 141

Jensen, M. P. 67

Johnson, N. E. 3

Jordan, C. P. 94

journaling 25
Joyal, C. C. 16
joyless play 153
Juliette (de Sade) 126
justice perspective 2
Justine (de Sade) 126

Kabiry, D. B. 96
Kaestle, C. E. 131
Kama Sutra 125
Karpman 141
Kauffman, M. 183
Kekatos, M. 74
Kelsey, K. 178
kinbaku 18–9
Kink Clinical Guidelines 180–2
kink community: educational
    opportunities and 104–9; munches
    and sloshes 103–4; overview
    103–11; research/educational
    organizations 106–9; virtual
    opportunities 109–10
kink overview 2–4
kink scenes *see* scenes
kink stigma *see* stigma
Kink-Affirming Practice (Goerlich)
    183–4
kink-affirming risk assessment
    158–63; *see also* assessment
kink-affirming treatment: best
    practices 184; clinicians 178–82;
    creating an affirming space
    188–90; effective interventions
    183–4; Kink Clinical Guidelines
    180–2; overview 191–2; power
    and control and 175–8; *see also*
    therapeutic relationship
kink-shaming 13
Kinsey, A. 95
Kinsey Institute 128, *128*
Kirschbaum, A. 130
Klaserner, M. 104
Klein, M. 136
Kleinplatz, P. 74

Kolmes, K 188, 189
Krauss, F. 141

lactophilia (breast milk fetish) 83
Langdridge, D. 50, 86
language 67–8, 141–3
Laqueur 130, 131
Lawson, J. 86
Leal, I. 131
Learn, J. R. 93
learning *see* educational
    opportunities
Lefevre, S. 162
legal factors: antisocial personalities
    and 72–3; discrimination and 72;
    kink-affirming treatment and
    185–8; laws 12; negotiation and
    117–8; risk assessment checklist
    173; total power exchange (TPE)
    and 42; *see also* criminal behaviors;
    problematic sexual behavior; risks
Lehmiller, J. 79, 87
Lengyell, M. 178
lesbian women 11; *see also*
    LGBTQIA+ community
Lester, P. E. 131
Levesque, R. J. 65
Levy, D. 101
Ley, D. 137
Lezos, A. M. 183, 184
LGBTQIA+ community: creating
    an affirming therapeutic space
    and 188–9; history of kink culture
    and 10–1; kink demographics and
    6; kink-affirming providers and
    179–80
Lilienfeld, S. O. 73
limits 114–5
Litam, S. 180, 188
Litsou, K. 135, 136
littles 80–1; *see also* age play
Lobbestael, J. 73
loneliness 137
Longman, III, T. 184

Longpre, N. 64
Lowrey, A. M. 163
Lucky, J. L. 90

Maczkowiack, J. 121
Maginn, P. 110
mainstream media 11–2
manslaughter 72
marginalized communities:
    kink-affirming providers and
    178–82; micro-aggressions and 1–2;
    therapeutic context and 176–7
Marie, C. 94
marks on the body 118–9, 122
Martinez, K. 74
masochism 4–5, 53–7; *see also*
    sadomasochism
masochistic altruism 69–70
Master 46
masturbation 2, 130–5, 136–7
Masuda, K. 96
materials fetishes 89, 90; *see also*
    fetishes and fetishistic desire
Mayo Clinic Staff 122
McArthur, N. 98
McClellan, S. 2, 183
McKee, A. 4, 135, 135, 152
McManus, M. A. 144
McNair, B. 11
mechanical bondage 19–21, 33–5;
    see also bondage
mediated sexuality 157
medical risks 117–8, 131;
    see also risks
Mehdizadeh-Zareanari, A. 96
Meibom, J. H. 10
mental health risks 131, 134–5
mental health services 72; *see also*
    kink-affirming treatment
mental illness: fetishes and fetishistic
    desire and 95–6; history of clinical
    biases 124–7; Kink Clinical
    Guidelines and 181, 183–4;
    objectophilia 97; out-of-control

sexual behavior (OCSB) and
    148–51; paraphilias and the DSM
    and 140–7; *see also* diagnosis;
    kink-affirming treatment
Merriam-Webster 27
Meyer, I. H. 88
micro-aggressions 1–2, 136, 161
middles 80–1; *see also* age play
Midori 16
minority communities 1–2, 12
Mokros, A. 64
Moll, A. 94, 95, 126
monogamish 139; *see also* ethical
    non-monogamy
Moors, A. 6
moral beliefs 138
Moran, M. 142
morning rituals 25; *see also* rituals
Morrens 6
Moser, C. 142, 188
motivation 67
munches 103–4; *see also*
    kink community
Murphy, C. 66
Murray, C. I. 78
mutual pleasure 150–1;
    see also pleasure
mythical creatures 87

National Coalition for Sexual
    Freedom (NCSF) 106–7, *107*,
    108, 185, 187
necrophilia 146
needs of each partner 153
negotiation: aftercare 120–3; 4Cs
    model and 167–8; goals/intentions
    and 112–4; intensity 113–5; limits
    114–5; marks and 118–9; overview
    112–23; physical touch and 116–7;
    RACK (Risk-Aware, Consensual
    Kink) and 164; risks and 117–8;
    safe words/gestures 115–6; scene
    details 116–7; "scenes" and 112;
    STI, disease, and pregnancy

protection and 118–9; total power exchange (TPE) and 42; trauma and trigger plans and 119; *see also* communication; consent
Nelson, T. 99
neurotransmitters 66
Nevard, I. 188
new paraphilic disorders 146–7
Newbold, S. 48
Newmahr, S. 38, 51, 112
Nichols, M. 69
Niedermeyer, T. 12
Nin, A. 70
Nitschke, J. 64
Nomis, A. 124, 125
non-consensual behavior: overview 129; pornography and 135–6; risk assessment checklist 173; when sexual behaviors are a problem 147–8; *see also* legal factors; problematic sexual behavior
nonexploitation 150
non-judgmental stance 160–2
non-monogamy: ethical non-monogamy 6, 138–40; without consent 138, 140
non-normative practices: history of clinical biases and 124–7; overview 1, 2–3; paraphilias and the DSM and 140–7; what counts as normal 128–30
normative practices 2–3, 124–30
numbness 34–5

Oakley, B. 68
object fetishes 89, 90, 91, 96–7; *see also* fetishes and fetishistic desire
Oddie, M. 13
Old Guard Leather 11
On the Cult of Fetish Gods (de Brosses) 93–4
On the Use of Flogging in Venereal Affairs 10, 12
120 Days of Sodom (de Sade) 126

Oneill, T. 2
online kink communities 110–1; *see also* kink community
online kink education 109–10
online porn 136–8; *see also* pornography
Oosterhuis, H. 95, 126
open relationships *see* ethical non-monogamy
operant conditioning 66
oppression 181
Oronowicz, W. 92
Osborn, C. A. 92
Osterheider, M. 64
otherwise specified paraphilic disorder 146
O'Toole, E. 72
out-of-control sexual behavior (OCSB) 148–51; *see also* problematic sexual behavior
Oyler, L. 3

Paarnio, M. 44
Paasonen, S. 77, 78–9, 80, 82
Pagan Bacchanalia 10
pain: authority exchange and 49; bondage and 34–5; idea of 53–4; purposeful pain 54–7; risk and benefits 74; sadism spectrum and 57–66; versus sensation 66–8; *see also* sadomasochism
paraphilia *see* fetishes and fetishistic desire
paraphilic disorders 101, 141–7, *143*
parental values 157; *see also* values
Patel, S. 66
pathological altruism 67–70
pathology: fetishes and fetishistic desire and 95; history of clinical biases and 124–7; paraphilias and the DSM and 140–7
Paulhus, D. L. 58
Peacock, S. 66
pedophilia 78, 90, 145

permission *see* consent; negotiation
personality 6–7, 43–5, 86
person-centered therapy 159–60
persuasion 169
pet play 84–7
Peterson, Z. 130
Pettyjohn, M. E. 177, 178
Phillips, J. 163
photography 10
physical risks 117–8, 133;
    see also risks
physical touch 116–7, 146, 173
Pittagora, D. 50, 183
place, idea of 2–3; *see also*
    Time+Place idea
play: cultural factors and 14;
    imaginative power exchange 77;
    predicament play 22; "scenes"
    111–2
pleasure: acceptance of 155; 4Ps
    model and 169; Kink Clinical
    Guidelines and 184; masturbation
    and 131–2; pain as 53; pleasure
    equity 2, 155; pleasure-seeking 54;
    principles of responsible sexual
    behavior and 150–1; purposeful
    pain and 54–5
Podolan, M. 158, 159
polyamory 6, 48, 139; *see also* ethical
    non-monogamy
pornography: BDSM portrayed in
    157; history of kink culture and 9,
    10; overview 135–8; what counts
    as normal and 128–9
power and power exchange:
    authority exchange and 36;
    caregiver kinks 78–84; cultural
    factors and 13–4; dominance and
    submission and 36–7, 38–43; 4Ps
    model and 168–9; history of kink
    culture and 9–10; imaginative
    power exchange 77; Kink Clinical
    Guidelines and 181; pet play 84–7;
    power theft 169; predicament

play and 22; protocols and 27–8;
    punishments and 30–2; purposeful
    pain and 54; risks and benefits
    49–51, 87–8; rituals and 25;
    rules and 24; sadomasochism
    and 70; safety and risks and 152,
    153–4; self-bondage and 19; sexual
    agency and 155; total power
    exchange (TPE) 38–43; in the
    treatment room 175–8; variations
    on D/s dynamics and 45–9
predicament play 22; *see also* bondage
pregnancy 118–9, 150
prejudice 88
Price, M. 67, 72
principles of responsible sexual
    behavior 150–1
privacy 42
private boundaries 153–4; *see also*
    boundaries
privilege 176–7, 178
problematic sexual behavior:
    ethical non-monogamy 138–40;
    masturbation 130–5; out-of-control
    sexual behavior (OCSB)
    148–51; paraphilias 140–7, *143*;
    pornography 135–8; what counts
    as normal and 128–30; when
    sexual behaviors are a problem
    147–51
professional education and training
    181–2
professional power 175–7; *see also*
    power and power exchange
pro-social sadism 59–60, 73, 76;
    see also sadism
protection 118–9
protocols 27–9; *see also* discipline
Prottle, Z. 34
providers 178–82; *see also*
    kink-affirming treatment
psychoeducation 67–8, 102, 160
psychological hedonism 53
psychological release 74

psychological risks 131, 134–5
psychopathy 73
Psychopatia Sexualis (Krafft-Ebing) 126
public boundaries 153–4; *see also* boundaries
public gatherings 104; *see also* munches
punishment and rewards protocols 28
punishment rituals 26; *see also* rituals
punishments 4, 15, 23, 28, 29–32; *see also* discipline
pup/puppy play 85–7; *see also* pet play
purpose, rituals and 25
purposeful pain 54–7; *see also* masochism; pain

Queer Liberation movement 11

race 12–3, 176–7; *see also* cultural factors
RACK (Risk-Aware, Consensual Kink) 164–6, 167, 168
Randall, A. 76, 121
rape 9, 72
Regnerus, M. 132
regression 81–2
Rehor, J. E. 48
rejection 161
rejection sensitivity 43
relational focus: overview 1–2; pet play and 86; power and control and 175; punishments and 28–9; purposeful pain and 55, 57; risk assessment checklist 171, 172, 173; sadomasochism and 74, 75; safety and risks and 155–6; *see also* relational risks
relational risks: masturbation and 133–4, 135; non-monogamy and 140; pornography and 136; risk assessment checklist 172, 173; *see also* relational focus; risks
relationship anarchy (RA) 139; *see also* ethical non-monogamy

religion: fetishes and fetishistic desire and 93; masturbation and 131, 132; pornography and 138; risk assessment checklist 172; rituals and 24
research/educational organizations 106–9
resilience 25, 74, 156
resistance 168–9
responsibility 30, 150–1
restraints 15, 17–9, 34–5; *see also* bondage
rewards 28
Rice, A. 11
Richardson, K. 101
Richters, J. 6, 68, 71
Riedel-Johnson, J. 4
riggers 35, 47
risks: aftercare and 122; assessment of 100, 158–63, 169–73; authority exchange and 49–51; bondage and discipline and 33–5; community framework and 163–9; conceptualizing through a kink-affirming lens 152–7; fetishes and fetishistic desire and 100–2; kink-affirming risk assessment and 158–63; marks and 118–9; masturbation and 133–5; negotiation and 117–8; non-monogamy and 140; risk assessment 100, 158–63, 169–73; risk assessment checklist 169–73; roleplay and 87–8; sadomasochism and 74–6; *see also* relational risks; safety
Ritchers 140
rituals 24–7, 28–9, 32; *see also* discipline
Robinson, W. 141
robosexuality 97–100; *see also* fetishes and fetishistic desire
roleplay: caregiver kinks 78–84; pet play 84–7; race play 12–3; risks

and benefits 87–8; variations on D/s dynamics and 48; *see also* imaginative power exchange
ropes 16, 17–9, 34–5; *see also* bondage
Rowland, D. L. 132
Rubin, G. 1
Rubin, L. 179
rules 23–4, 28–9; *see also* discipline
Rulof, P. 78, 79
rumination 129; *see also* problematic sexual behavior

sadism 4–5, 53–4, 57–66; *see also* sadomasochism
sadistic personality disorder (SPD) 65–6, 72–4
sadomasochism: adult babies/diaper lovers and 84; authority exchange and 38; conflict resolution and 32; differential diagnostics 68–74; discipline and 15; history of kink culture and 9–10; idea of pain and 53–4; overview 5, 52; pain versus sensation and 66–8; purposeful pain and 54–7; risk and benefits 74–6; sadism spectrum and 57–66; safety and risks and 153; sexual sadism disorder and 65
safe words/gestures 115–6
safety: authority exchange and 49–51; bondage and discipline and 33–5; community framework and 163–9; conceptualizing through a kink-affirming lens 152–7; creating an affirming therapeutic space and 188–90; educational events and 105; kink-affirming risk assessment and 158–63; principles of responsible sexual behavior and 150–1; problematic sexual behavior and 128–9; punishments and 31; risk assessment checklist 169–73; total

power exchange (TPE) and 42; *see also* risks
Sagarin, B. 50, 62–3, 74, 108
Saketopoulou, A. 70
Salmon, L. 178
Samois 11
Sand, L. 183
Sandnabba, N. K. 71
scenes: aftercare 120–3; consent and 167; cultural factors and 14; details of 116–7; goals/intentions and 113–4; intensity of 113–5; limits 114–5; marks and 118–9; negotiation and 111–2, 112–23; overview 111–3; physical touch and 116–7; risks and 117–8; safe words/gestures 115–6; STI, disease, and pregnancy protection and 118–9; trauma and trigger plans and 119
Schnider, A. 172
Schori, A. 49
Schweitzer 121
Science of BDSM Lab 108, *108*
Scorolli, C. 92
Scott, C. 70
screentime control 41
security 50
self-acceptance 154–5
self-bondage 19, 33–4; *see also* bondage
self-esteem 74
self-harm 70–2, 133
self-sacrificing 69
sensation: authority exchange and 49; bondage and 16; exchange of 5; fetishes and 89; masturbation and 132; mechanical bondage and 20–1; pain and 65–8; purposeful pain and 54–5; sadism spectrum and 66; sadomasochism and 74; sensory deprivation 17, 30
service expectations protocols 28
sessions 111–3; *see also* scenes

Severe Sexual Sadism Scale (SSSS) 63–5
sex toys 117
sex-affirming treatment *see* kink-affirming treatment
sexual addiction 138, 155; *see also* problematic sexual behavior
sexual agency *see* agency
sexual assault 185–7; *see also* criminal behaviors
sexual control 40
sexual masochism disorder 144–5
sexual sadism disorder 57–9, 63–5, 145; *see also* sadism
sexually transmitted infections 118–9, 150
shame: boundaries and 154; masturbation and 131, 132, 135, 137; paraphilic disorders and 144–5; pornography and 136; problematic sexual behavior and 130; sadomasochism and 69, 76; safety and risks and 154–5
shared values 150; *see also* values
Sheff, E. 138–9
Sheppard, E. 56, 57
Shibari 18–9
Shorter, E. 126, 144
Shulman, J. L. 131
Simone, M. 81
Simula, B. L. 45, 46
Siwak, M. 92
skill-building education 35, 105; *see also* educational opportunities
Slagstad, K. 163
slave 46
slavery 9
Sleeping Beauty Trilogy (Roquelaure) 11
Sloan, K. 183
sloshes 103–4; *see also* kink community
social control 42

social factors: privilege and 176–7; risk assessment checklist 172; risks and benefits of authority exchange and 50; rituals and 24; stigma and 148; values and 157
social gatherings 103–4; *see also* kink community
sociocultural norms 149–50
socio-political power 176–7
Solitary Sex (Laqueur) 130
Song, X. 100
Speciale, M. 180, 188
spreader bars 20–1; *see also* bondage
Sprott, R. A. 6, 48, 76, 120, 180
SSC (safe, sane, and consensual) 164, 165–6, 167
St. Andrews Cross 21
Stein, D. 164
Steinmetz, C. 110
stereotypes 43, 49, 124–7; *see also* stigma
Stevenson, D. 10
stigma: boundaries and 154; Kink Clinical Guidelines and 181, 182; kink-affirming risk assessment and 158; kink-affirming treatment and 180, 188–9; language of pain and 67; masturbation and 131; overview 1–2; paraphilias and 141, 143–4; pornography and 135–6; problematic sexual behavior and 130; purposeful pain and 57; roleplay and 88; sadism spectrum and 59; SSC (safe, sane, and consensual) and 164; when sexual behaviors are a problem 148; *see also* stereotypes
Stock, W. 188
Stone, D. 176, 177
The Story of O 11
stress: masturbation and 132; risk assessment checklist 173; risks and

benefits of authority exchange and 50; sadomasochism and 74

Stromberg, J. 73

subjective wellbeing 43; *see also* wellbeing

submission: adult babies/diaper lovers and 84; authority exchange 36–8; overview 4–5; personality traits and 43–5; power exchange and 38–43; risks and benefits of authority exchange and 49–51; variations on D/s dynamics 45–9

submissives: authority exchange and 37–8; kink demographics and 6; predicament play and 22; rituals and 25–6; self-bondage and 19; total power exchange (TPE) and 38–43; variations on D/s dynamics 45–9

substance use: bondage and discipline and 34; fetishes and fetishistic desire and 96; risk assessment checklist 173; risks and benefits of authority exchange and 49

surface consent 167; *see also* consent

Swartzendruber, A. 149

swinging 138–9; *see also* ethical non-monogamy

switch 37, 45–9; *see also* Dominants; submissives

Switch, G. 164–5

task-based rituals 25–6; *see also* rituals

Tatum, A. K. 12

taxonomy of kink **7–8**

technosexuality 97–100, 101

teledildonics 97–100; *see also* fetishes and fetishistic desire

telephone scatologia 147

Tell Me What You Want (Lehmiller) 87

therapeutic relationship 61–2, 159, 175–8, 191–2; *see also* kink-affirming treatment

therapists 178–82; *see also* kink-affirming treatment

Thomas, L. 110

Three Essays on the Theory of Sexuality (Freud) 126–7

Tiidenberg, K. 78–9, 80, 82

time control 42

Time+Place idea 2–4, 89, 96, 192

tops 22, 45–9, 153

total power exchange (TPE) 38–43; *see also* power and power exchange

Toth, J. 60, 62, 72, 75–6

touch, physical 116–7, 146, 173

Townsend, E. 71

Tracey, I. 67

Trammell, A. 14

transvestic disorder 145

trauma: fetishes and fetishistic desire and 96; Kink Clinical Guidelines and 180, 183–4; kink-affirming risk assessment and 159; objectophilia and 97; risk assessment checklist 171; self-harm and 71–2; trauma and trigger plans and 119

Treating Out of Control Sexual Behavior (Braun-Harvey & Vigorito) 148–50

treatment, kink-affirming *see* kink-affirming treatment

trigger plans 119

Tupper, P. 10

Turley, E. 38, 74

Turvey, B. 69

Twist, M. 98

Udodiong, I. 3

unspecified paraphilic disorder 146

urolagnia (urine fetish) 83, 147

validation 162–3

values 150, 157

van Assen, M. 43–4, 71

van der Beek, S. 110
Vandiver, D. 66, 73
Vatsyayana 125
Venus in Furs (von Sacher-Masoch) 126
Vess, J. 66
Vick, M. 63
Victoria Department of Health 171–2
Vigorito, M. 147, 148–50, 151
Vilkin, E. 48
violence 181
virtual kink education 110–1
virtual reality (VR) 98, 99; *see also* digisexuality
virtue 55
visual erotica 3–4
von Krafft-Ebing, R. 94, 95, 125–6
von Sacher-Masoch, L. 126
voyeurism 146, 173
vulnerability: bondage 21; bondage and 16; self-bondage and 19; trauma and trigger plans and 119

Waldura, J. F. 49, 50, 188
wardrobe protocols 28
Watts-Jones, D. 177
Webster, C. 104
Weisel-Barth, J. 96
Weisman, C. 16
Weiss, M. D. 104
wellbeing: dominance and submission and 43; Kink Clinical Guidelines and 181; kink-affirming risk assessment and 158; risks and benefits of authority exchange and 50–1; sadomasochism and 74
Wellings, K. 125
Wertheimer, A. 149–50
Westen, D. 61
Wiech, K. 67
Wignall, L. 85, 110
wild animals, pet play and 87
Williams, D. 6, 38–9, 167
Wiseman, J. 16, 34
Wisemeijer, A. 43–4, 71
Wood, H. 59
work/career control 42
World Health Organization 180
World War II 10–1, 141
Worthen, M. G. 65
Wright, S. 101, 142

Xygalatas, D. 57

Yager, J. 161
Yakeley, J. 59
Yost, M. R. 6

Zambelli, L. 110
Zamboni, B. 83, 84, 96
Zenilman, J. M. 149
Zhang, K. T 3
zoophilia 84–5, 146

Printed in the United States
by Baker & Taylor Publisher Services